Fundamental aspects of infection prevention and control

Other titles in the series include
Fundamental Aspects of Long-Term Conditions
Fundamental Aspects of Palliative Care Nursing 2nd Edition
Fundamental Aspects of Research for Nurses
Fundamental Aspects of Finding Information
Fundamental Aspects of Pain Assessment

Coming soon
Fundamental Aspects of Legal, Ethical & Professional Issues 2nd edition
Fundamental Aspects of Ophthalmic Nursing

Series editor
Dr John Fowler

Note

Healthcare practice and knowledge are constantly changing and developing as new research and treatments, changes in procedures, drugs and equipment become available.

The author and publishers have, as far as is possible, taken care to confirm that the information complies with the latest standards of practice and legislation.

Fundamental aspects of infection prevention and control

Edited by

Vinice Thomas

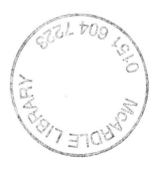

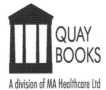

QUAY
BOOKS

A division of MA Healthcare Ltd

Quay Books Division, MA Healthcare Ltd, St Jude's Church, Dulwich Road, London
SE24 0PB

British Library Cataloguing-in-Publication Data
A catalogue record is available for this book

© MA Healthcare Limited 2011
ISBN-10: 1-85642-415-4;
ISBN-13: 978-1-85642-415-8

Edited by Jessica Anderson

Printed by CLE, Huntingdon, Cambridgeshire

Contents

List of contributors   *vi*

Foreword   *viii*

1   Introduction   1
   Vinice Thomas

Section 1: Understanding infection   7

2   Infectious agents   9
   David Tucker

3   Means of transmission of infectious agents   27
   Sheila Loveridge

Section 2: Prevention and control   45

4   Staff health   47
   Dorothy N Chakani

5   Environmental hygiene   71
   Emily Hoban

6   Decontamination of reusable surgical instruments   97
   Louise Hodgson

7   Protective measures   113
   Andrea Denton and Christine Berry

8   Special precautions   135
   Carole Hallam and Sandra Mogford

Section 3: Management and treatment   153

9   Management of invasive devices   155
   Annette Jeanes

10   Caring for an infected patient   181
   Rachel Ben Salem

11   Antibacterial agents and their role in infection control   193
   Christianne Micallef

12   Infection prevention and control:
   Roles and resposibilities   223
   Vinice Thomas

Index   237

List of contributors

Rachel Ben Salem BSc(Hons) Microbiology, Dip(Infection Control), PGCert(Academic Practice) is Senior Infection Control Nurse, Kings College Hospital NHS Foundation Trust, London

Christine Berry RGN is Infection Prevention and Control Nurse, Calderdale and Huddersfield NHS Foundation Trust

Dorothy N Chakani Dip(HEN), CertSpmic, RGN is Senior Infection Control Practitioner, West Sussex Health, West Sussex

Andrea Denton MA, MSc, BSc(Hons), DPSN, RNT, RGN is Infection Prevention and Control Nurse, Calderdale and Huddersfield NHS Foundation Trust

Carole Hallam MSc, BSc(Hons), CertHeEd, RGN, RMN is Assistant Director of Infection Prevention and Control, Calderdale and Huddersfield NHS Foundation Trust. She is also Branch Co-ordinator for the Infection Prevention Society. Currently Associate Portfolio Manager for the Department of Health National Healthcare-Associated Infection Team

Emily Hoban is Assistant General Manager, Specialist Services, Southport and Ormskirk Hospitals NHS Trust. She is an accredited trainer for the Chartered Institute of Environmental Health. Currently Cleaning Specialist for the Department of Health National Healthcare-Associated Infection Team

Louise Hodgson BSc, Cert IC (University of Leeds), RGN is Team Leader, Infection Prevention Team, Wakefield Distict Comunity Healthcare Services

Annette Jeanes MSc, Dip(N), Dip(IC), RN is Director of Infection Prevention and Control, Consultant Nurse Infection Control, University College London NHS Foundation Trust

Sheila Loveridge BSc, RGN, Dip HEd, Dip IC, MSc (Public Health) is Consultant Nurse, Infection Control, Western Sussex Hospitals NHS Trust, Worthing

Christianne Micallef BPharm(Hons), MPhil, PhD, MRPharmS is Lead Specialist Antimicrobial Pharmacist, Queen Elizabeth Hospital Kings Lynn NHS Trust. Currently Specialist Project Support Practitioner for Antimicrobial Prescribing for the Department of Health National Healthcare-Associated Infection Team

Sandra Mogford DipHE, RN (Adult) is Infection Prevention and Control Nurse, Calderdale and Huddersfield NHS Foundation Trust

Vinice Thomas MBA, BSc(Hons), PGDipEd, RGN is Assistant Director of Nursing/Clinical Governance and Director of Infection Prevention and Control, Harrow PCT. Currently Portfolio Manager for the Department of Health National Healthcare-Associated Infection Team

David Tucker BSc (Infection Prevention) is Deputy Director of Infection Prevention and Control, Guy's and St Thomas' NHS Foundation Trust, London and Honorary Lecturer, King's College London

Foreword

Infection prevention is a responsibility everyone shares, and the reduction of healthcare-associated infections (HCAI) remains a duty of every NHS organisation. Good hand hygiene, high standards of cleanliness, prudent antimicrobial prescribing and effective patient screening are all vitally important in the fight against HCAIs.

There has already been a significant reduction across the NHS in some HCAIs, specifically MRSA and *Clostridium difficile*. However, there remains capacity for these and other infections to be reduced further.

Within the pages of this book, you will find information and guidance, with tools and examples of successful infection prevention and control practice. These will help you, your organisation, and patients and visitors to play a part in reducing infections. By reducing infections, we can save lives and reduce the unnecessary pain and suffering caused to patients, their families and loved ones.

Patients and service users expect high standards of safety and cleanliness in their care. Reducing HCAI rates and communicating these results will help those you care for have confidence in the service you provide and reduce their fears and anxieties. The prevention and control of infections is not just a professional duty but also a clinical and managerial responsibility.

HCAIs cost the health service around £1 billion per year. In addition, evidence suggests that service users with MRSA bacteraemia spend on average an additional 10 days in hospital, whilst those with *Clostridium difficile* spend an additional 21 days in hospital. Reducing HCAIs helps the NHS make the most of its resources and deliver more for its users.

All healthcare staff have a duty and responsibility to provide an environment within which clean, safe care can be delivered. Reducing infection improves care and overall health outcomes for patients.

Find out what you and your organisation can do to help tackle infections.

Professor Janice Stevens CBE

CHAPTER 1

Introduction

Vinice Thomas

Purpose

The purpose of this chapter is to set the context for infection prevention and control within health and social care settings, and to provide a brief overview of the book.

Learning outcomes

By the end of this chapter, you will have learned:

- The importance of infection prevention and control.
- The key components of effective infection prevention and control.
- How to use this book as a tool for personal and professional development.

Introduction

Infection control is an exciting and rewarding aspect of patient care which has evolved over the past decade. It is exciting because of the ongoing medical advances and discoveries that have helped to eradicate or control diseases which, in previous years, would have inevitably resulted in fatalities. It is rewarding because, through good stewardship of antibiotics, consistent application of good hand hygiene, and good management of medical devices and other elements of patient care, recovery from life-threatening infections is possible. Job satisfaction for many is found in the knowledge that one has contributed to a positive outcome be it a speedy recovery or a peaceful and dignified end of life.

In the quest to deliver high standards of care, healthcare workers have strived to overcome barriers to quality care, with the reduction of infections being a key challenge. One commonly held view was that infections were inevitable when patients were admitted to hospital for treatment. As a result significant reductions in healthcare associated infections (HCAIs) had, until recently, been considered to be an unachievable goal. By 2008, there was a significant reduction in methicillin-resistant *Staphylococcus aureus* (MRSA) and an improvement in *Clostridium difficile* rates of infection (Department of Health 2008a). Although these two infections received

1

a great deal of focus and media attention, it was clear that healthcare organisations were also grappling with other HCAIs. However, lessons learnt from tackling MRSA were transferable to other infections. For instance, the elements of care found to be effective in reducing MRSA and *Clostridium difficile* rates, such as good hand hygiene, were applicable to all of the other infections. Indeed some hospitals reported an improvement in other HCAIs as a result of improved practices for MRSA.

Although the causes and management of infections are multifaceted and at times complex, national and global work on reducing HCAIs has highlighted some key factors that can achieve significant results. This involves the consistent application of a number of actions that together make the reduction of infections achievable. These include the appropriate use of antibiotics, management of invasive medical devices, and cleanliness of the environment, to mention but a few. However, the activities must be applied consistently by all staff. This means there is no room for deviating from what is known to be best practice without a real danger of harm to patients.

In 1859, Florence Nightingale, the founder of modern nursing, stated:

It may seem a strange principle to enunciate as the very first requirement in a hospital that it should do the sick no harm.

(Nightingale 1992)

This can be applied to every setting where care is given to patients or clients, be it in the community, in care or nursing homes, in acute settings within busy wards, or specialist areas such as intensive care units or burns units. Despite various competing priorities, it is important that patients/service users receive care that has no negative effect. As Professor Sir Ian Kennedy expressed aptly:

Safety cannot ever be allowed to play second fiddle to other objectives that may emerge from time to time…it is the first objective.

(Healthcare Commission 2006)

Infection control must be at the heart of safe care, and should be an integral part of daily activities undertaken by staff. No staff member should be excluded from contributing to the control of infections (Healthcare Commission 2007).

Throughout the history of health and social care, there have been incidents where outbreaks of infections have had a devastating effect on individuals and their families. This becomes even more devastating when analysis of the outbreaks has shown incidences where the infection may have been prevented or the spread minimised. More recently, incidents such as outbreaks of infections in various hospitals have highlighted the far reaching effect poor infection control can have on patients, their relatives and the local community (Healthcare Commission 2006, 2009). In some cases, patients experienced untold suffering resulting in extended hospital stays, others died. The local community, once made aware of this by extensive media coverage, can begin to lose confidence in its local NHS trust.

There are many lessons that can be learnt from these incidents which are relevant to the fundamental aspects of infection prevention and control that, when applied, can significantly reduce the likelihood of infections and outbreaks within homes, clinical areas, healthcare organisations and communities. This book will cover some of these key aspects of care. Drawing on invaluable tools and lessons from the Department of Health (2008b), this book aims to help equip staff with the skills to reduce avoidable healthcare-associated infections.

Outline of the book

This book is divided into three sections:

1. Understanding infection.
2. Prevention and control.
3. Management and treatment.

Understanding infections

The first section begins with an introduction to how infectious agents operate; *Chapter 2* looks at the physiology and classification of these agents and provides a basis for further study into this complex subject. Building on this, *Chapter 3* looks at how these agents are transmitted to others. This enables readers to identify key routes and the subsequent preventative actions that can be taken to break the chain of transmission.

Prevention and control

The next section focuses on the actions health and social care workers can take to prevent and control the spread of infections. *Chapter 4* examines the responsibility of staff to ensure they are fit to practice. The importance of undergoing the necessary precautions to safeguard their health and well-being and ultimately that of their patients is emphasised. National patient surveys have shown the importance patients place on the appearance of the environment within which they will be nursed. This has often been key when patients are identifying the hospital of their choice. Issues surrounding hygiene, cleanliness of the environment and the use of protective measures are explored in *Chapters 5, 6, 7* and *8*.

Management and treatment

The final section of the book discusses the management and care of patients. There are many medical procedures and devices which, although instrumental in improving patient care, can become a route for infection if not managed safely. *Chapter 9* examines the management of invasive medical devices and the general care required for infected patients. Treatment and procedures are discussed in *Chapter 10*.

Good antibiotic stewardship has been considered one of the most important aspects of treatment because of the rising number of microorganisms resistant to 'mainstream' antimicrobials. *Chapter 11* provides a detailed review of antimicrobials.

Building on all the preceding chapters, the final chapter highlights the role and responsibilities of staff to deliver the infection prevention and control agenda.

Psychological effects of infection

Throughout the book, mention is made of the importance of information and reassurance for patients. The psychological effect of infection must not be underestimated or overlooked amidst the busyness of treatment and management. Patients and their relatives may experience the stigma of being infected and placed in isolation. A common complaint of patients is the feeling of loneliness when they have had to be isolated and the sense of rejection they feel when they are cared for by staff wearing protective masks, aprons and gloves. Loss of human contact can have an adverse effect on patients.

Furthermore, the inability to communicate or understand instructions given around infection prevention and control due to a medical disorder, such as Alzheimer's syndrome, neurological conditions or language barriers, can perpetuate anxiety and fear of the unknown. It is important therefore that patients/ service users are provided with information in a variety of ways to enable them to understand the guidance for preventing cross-infection. These problems can be overcome by providing clear information, e.g. patient leaflets translated into different languages, or visual aids and guidance, and psychological support, such as reassurance and comfort.

Study tools

Each chapter provides opportunities for readers to focus on key points, or to undertake reflective or explorative activities in order to apply and improve knowledge. Readers are advised to consider the use of a reflective journal or a similar tool to capture learning. This will be invaluable for sharing with a supervisor within the clinical setting or place of study.

External agencies

At the time of writing there have been significant changes in the political and economical climate within health and social care in Britain. As a result, some of the external agencies referred to in this book, such as the National Patient Safety Agency, will undergo changes to their roles and functions. However, it is envisaged that healthcare organisations will continue to build on the achievements gained to provide safe care for patients.

Summary

This chapter has set the context within which healthcare workers strive to deliver quality care. It has looked at some of the challenges around the infection prevention and control agenda, and at how applying lessons learnt from outbreaks of infection is key to reducing the likelihood of a recurrence. The chapter provided a brief overview of the fundamental issues of infection prevention and control, and looked at how best the reader can achieve the learning outcomes in order to be well equipped to contribute to this important aspect of care.

In the next chapter we will begin to understand infectious agents and how they operate.

References

Department of Health (2008a) *Clean safe care: Reducing infections and saving lives.* Gateway ref: 9278. Department of Health, London

Department of Health (2008b) *The Health and Social Care Act: Code of Practice for health and adult social care on the prevention and control of infections and related guidance.* Gateway 13072. Department of Health, London

Healthcare Commission (2006) *Investigation of outbreaks of Clostridium difficile at Stoke Mandeville Hospital.* Buckinghamshire Hospitals NHS Trust. Buckingham

Healthcare Commission (2007) *Healthcare associated infections: What else can the NHS do?* Healthcare Commission, London

Healthcare Commission, (2009) *Investigation into Mid-Staffordshire NHS Foundation Trust*. Healthcare Commission, London

Nightingale F (1992) *Notes on nursing: What it is, and what it is not* (Commemorative edn). J.B. Lippincott, Philadelphia

Section 1

Understanding infection

CHAPTER 2

Infectious agents

David Tucker

Purpose

The purpose of this chapter is to give an overview of infectious agents which may have an adverse effect on the health and well-being of patients, clients and staff. We will look at their classification, the types of infections they may cause and the growth cycle or microorganisms.

Learning outcomes

By the end of the chapter, you will have learned:

- How to classify a microorganism based on its characteristics.
- Different types of organisms such as bacteria, viruses and fungi.
- The phases of the growth cycle.
- Examples of infections that microorganism can cause.

Introduction

An understanding of microorganisms is essential to underpinning informed practice in infection prevention and control. This chapter provides a basic introduction to the speciality area, but readers are strongly urged to undertake further reading to gain a deeper understanding.

Simplistically, microbiology is the study of organisms that are too small to be seen individually by the naked eye, and thus require the use of specialist equipment, i.e. microscopes, to be able to visualise them. Colonies of microorganisms on growth media, e.g. *Staphylococcus aureus*, are visible to the naked eye. However, this is not their normal environment or appearance.

The presence of microorganisms was first demonstrated by Antony Van Leeuwnhoek in the 17th century using a microscope (Wilson 2006). However, it was not until the mid-19th century, as a consequence of the work by Louis Pasteur and Robert Koch, amongst others, who identified the association of bacteria with infection, that the association between microorganisms and disease developed (Mims et al 1998). In 1884, in his treatise on *Mycobacterium tuberculosis* and tuberculosis

Koch postulated that key elements were necessary for bacteria to be associated with infection. Latterly, whilst these postulates form the bedrock of the understanding of bacterial infection, they have been demonstrated as being too narrow in their definition, although not surprisingly since the science has advanced.

In summary the postulates are (Brooks et al 2001):

- The microorganism shall be found in all cases of the disease in question and its distribution in the body shall be in accordance with the lesions observed.
- The microorganism shall be grown in pure culture *in vitro* (or outside the body of the host) for several generations.
- When such a pure culture is inoculated into susceptible animal species, the typical disease must result.
- The microorganism must again be isolated from the lesions of such experimentally produced disease.

Whilst Florence Nightingale's understanding and acceptance of micro-organisms in the role of infection may be debated (McInnes 1990), she based her hygienic standards on cleanliness, good ventilation and sanitation (Nightingale 1860) which would have had an impact on the risk of cross-infection and contamination. Dr John Snow, of the Broad Street pump fame, demonstrated, through the epidemiological study of mortality related to cholera (Hempel 2007), the association of cause and effect from a demonstrable source of contamination.

Microorganisms are ubiquitous, that is they can be found anywhere and everywhere. The actions or activity of the majority of organisms is such that they will not have a direct impact, and are unlikely to cause disease to man. In fact some organisms will have a beneficial impact, whilst a relatively small number of others will be pathogenic; that is they are capable of causing disease/infection and death in man. To become pathogenic the organisms have to be able to enter the body and cause an adverse reaction that is potentially harmful and capable of overcoming the individual's immune system to cause disease. Most areas of the

---

Key points

- *Pathogenic* organisms are organisms that are capable of causing disease/infection
- *Commensal* organisms are organism that live within the body but cause no harm and may be beneficial to the host

body are colonised by bacteria that live within that environment, causing no harm, and may have a beneficial relationship with the 'host'; these organisms are known as commensals. However, should these organisms be transferred to other parts of the body, e.g. through breaks in the skin, they may cause infection, for example, *Escherichia coli,* a commensal of the gut, is a significant cause of ascending urinary tract infections in young girls, primarily because of the close proximity of the anus to the urethra.

This chapter consists of the following sections:

- Classification and types of organisms.
- The growth cycle of microorganisms.
- Examples of infectious organisms and the infections they may cause.

Classification and types of organisms

Organisms are principally classified according to their characteristics, and fall into four main groupings:

- Bacteria
- Fungi
- Protozoa
- Viruses.

All living organisms are comprised of one of two types of cell: eukaryotic or prokaryotic (Mims et al 1998). Eukaryotic cells are complex arrangements and are the building blocks of many living structures, including animals, plants, fungi and protozoa. Within their arrangements eukaryotic cells undertake many functions within the complete structure. Prokaryotic cells are simpler structures, forming single-celled organisms, such as bacteria. *See Figure 2.1.*

Bacteria

Bacteria are classified according to three main characteristics (Wilson 2006): the cell wall's ability to stain (for visual recognition); the shape of the cell; and use of oxygen.

- *Gram stain*: In the 19th century Christian Gram, a Danish bacteriologist, developed a technique of staining microorganisms to enable them to be

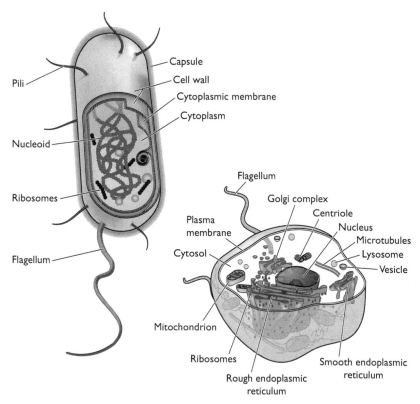

Figure 2.1. Prokaryotic cell structure. (left) and eukaryotic cell structure (right).

seen under a microscope (being thin walled, bacteria are transparent and not easily seen). When a blue dye (usually crystal violet) and iodine are applied to the bacteria and retained by the cell wall when washed with acetone, the bacteria will appear dark blue under the microscope. These cells are known as Gram-positive bacteria. Those bacteria that have a non-absorbent cell wall and do not absorb the crystal violet are described as Gram-negative, and to enable them to be seen under the microscope they have to have a second dye, usually safranin, applied (red in colour).

- *Shape (morphology)*: Once visualised, bacteria are described according to their appearance or shape (see *Figure 2.2*):
  - Cocci are round.
  - Bacilli are rod-shaped.
  - Spirochetes are spiral.

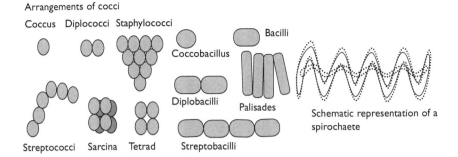

Figure 2.2. Different shapes of bacteria.

- *Oxygen*: Bacteria fall into one of three categories according to their relationship with oxygen
  - *Obligate aerobes* require oxygen to live or grow.
  - *Obligate anaerobes* are unable to survive in an oxygen environment.
  - *Facultative anaerobes* are able to grow with or without oxygen.

Spore-forming bacteria

Spore-forming bacteria are so called because they form bacterial spores. These bacteria have the capability to survive hostile environments through the enveloping of DNA particles within a cell membrane which may serve to protect them against hostile conditions, and, when circumstances improve, enable them to regenerate into viable organisms.

Examples of the different types of bacteria and their characteristics are outlined in *Table 1.1* (Brooks et al 2001).

The cell walls of bacteria are formed of either peptidoglycan (carbohydrates and amino acids) and are Gram-positive, or a combination of phospholipids and peptidoglycan (Gram-negative). In Gram-negative organisms the outer layer contains lipopolysaccharides, which may produce endotoxins and be harmful to the host. Bacteria reproduce by a process of binary fission, that is, the cell divides to form two daughter cells. Most cells are incapable of independent movement, however, some Gram-negative organisms, e.g. *Escherichia coli* and *Pseudomonas* have flagella on their cell walls which act like propellers so that they can move towards nutrients.

Continued survival of bacteria depends on

- A continuous supply of nutrients, including carbon and nitrogen.

Table 1.1. Types of bacteria

Shape	Gram stain	Oxygen requirement	Examples	Common site of occurrence
Cocci	Positive	Aerobic	• *Staphylococci:* aureus epidermidis	• Skin • Mucous membranes
Cocci	Positive	Facultative anaerobes	• *Streptococci:* Group A (pyogenes) Group B	• Throat and skin • Intestine and vagina
Bacilli	Negative	Aerobic	• *Escherichia coli* • *Klebsiella* spp.	• Gut
Bacilli	Negative	Anaerobic	• *Bacteroides fragilis*	• Gut
Bacilli (acid fast)	Positive (special stain required)	Aerobic	• *Mycobacterium tuberculosis*	• Lung
Spirochetes	Special stain required	? Aerobic	*Treponema pallidum*	• Skin • Mucous membranes

- Moisture, particularly Gram-negative organisms which will thrive in damp environments but die rapidly if dried out (Gram-positive organisms can survive for extended periods in dry conditions).
- Oxygen, as described above.
- Temperature, those organisms that are most closely associated with humans operate most effectively at body temperature.
- Acidity, most bacteria prefer a neutral solution, although others can survive at the extremes of the pH range.

Fungi

Fungi are plants and are eukaryotic cells. Fungi are primarily divided into yeasts and filamentous fungi. Yeasts are round or oval cells that reproduce by budding from division of a parent cell. Filamentous fungi produce filaments or hyphae that can branch out to form a mesh or mass, called mycelium (Mims et al 1998).

> ## Key points
>
> - Microorganisms are not normally visible to the naked eye, and to examine them in a laboratory they need to be seen under a microscope
> - Not all microorganisms possess the potential to cause harm to humans, and may be beneficial to the host
> - Specific organisms may be associated with particular body systems
> - All microorganisms have specific requirements to live and reproduce; knowledge of these requirements may help to combat potential infections

Protozoa

Protozoa are much larger than bacteria and are eukaryotic cells. They may obtain nutrients through the ingestion of organic material, and may be motile with either flagella or cilia (Mims et al 1998).

Viruses

Unlike the preceding organisms viruses are not cells, but are comprised of nucleic acid (DNA or RNA) surrounded by a capsid (protein coat), and as such are obligate parasites, i.e. they require a host cell in which to survive and reproduce. The virus normally will destroy the host cell, but then move on to infect an adjacent cell (Mims et al 1998).

The growth cycle of microorganisms

The determination of the survival of microorganisms is dictated primarily by the availability of nutrients. Cellular growth depends on the availability of nutrients; a shortage ultimately leading to death. The speed with which colonies will expand depends on the availability of nutrients, environmental factors and the organism itself, with doubling of cells primarily determined by the reproductive rate of the organism. In Brooks et al (2001) the growth curve of microbial cells clearly demonstrates the phases as a predictive process (see *Figure 2.3*):

- The lag phase (A and B): Cells adapt to their new environment.
- The exponential phase (C and D): Cells are being produced at a constant

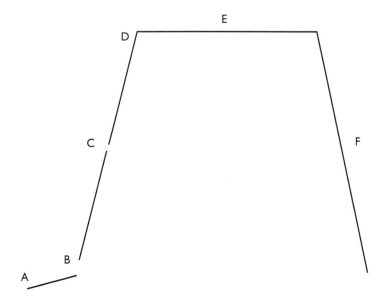

Figure 2.3. Growth pattern of microbial cells.

rate until nutrients become depleted or toxic metabolites accumulate and cause growth inhibition.

• The stationary phase (E): Exhaustion of nutrients or the accumulation of toxins causes growth to cease; although some new cells may continue to develop, the viable count remains constant

• The death phase (F): This occurs after the stationary phase and continues until the position is reversed or the colonies are destroyed. In reality small numbers of cells will survive and, with the introduction of fresh nutrients, growth will reoccur.

Examples of infections

The following section examines some infections which are found in healthcare settings (Mims et al 1998). Although specific emphasis is placed on bacterial infections as these are the most common infections, a brief overview of fungal and viral infections is also provided. Readers are advised to undergo further study of these latter infections if required.

Bacterial infection

The following are examples of the more commonly occurring bacteria that may cause infections, particularly within the healthcare setting.

Gram-positive cocci

Staphylococci are Gram-positive organisms that form irregular groupings, often referred to as resembling bunches of grapes. Some are normal colonisers of the skin and mucous membranes, whilst others cause suppurative infections, abscesses, other pyogenic infections, septicaemias and death. The two main staphylococcal infections are *Staphylococcus aureus* and *Staphylococcus epidermidis* (Brooks et al 2001).

- *Staphylococcus aureus* is commonly found colonising normal skin sites, including the nose, axillae, groin and perineum. Given an opportunity to enter the skin it can cause significant infection, ranging from superficial skin infections, including boils, impetigo and abscesses, to more serious infections, including wound infections, osteomyelitis, septicaemia and endocarditis. Some strains are capable of producing toxins which may cause a range of illnesses, including toxic shock syndrome, or extensive tissue necrosis, e.g. Panton-Valentine Leukocidin *S. aureus* or food poisoning. Public awareness of *S. aureus* is high because of the resistant strain MRSA. *S. aureus* is associated with both hospital and community acquired infections irrespective of its resistance pattern. However, the organism is known for its ability to acquire resistance to the penicillin group of antibiotics, primarily through the production of the enzyme β-lactamase, which interrupts the activity of the antibiotic.
- *Staphylococcus epidermidis* colonises the skin and is known as a coagulase-negative *Staphylococcus*. Coagulase is an enzyme that clots plasma through reacting with a factor in the plasma, and is a feature of *S. aureus*. Coagulase-negative staphylococci have assumed significance through their affinity to plastic or metal devices implanted in the body, including intravenous catheters and joint and valve prostheses, which, given their usage in medicine, can be a significant problem. Coagulase-negative staphylococci are commonly associated with septicaemia.

Streptococci are Gram-positive cocci that form into pairs or chains (Brooks et al 2001). Streptococci, a broad group of bacteria, are members of the normal human flora, and only cause infection when they become translocated to areas where they do not normally occur, or from person to person. However, they may be associated with a range of significant infections. These bacteria are classified through their morphology, their appearance on blood agar (haemolytic), serological markers of the cell wall, and other factors. The cell wall of β-haemolytic streptococci produce an antigen and are classified into serological groupings, known as the Lancefield groups (A to S). The action of haemolysis is most notable in necrotising fasciitis (primarily associated with Group A streptococci, although other organisms are implicated), in which the release of exotoxins causes widespread necrosis of soft tissues. Four streptococci infections are considered here:

- Group A streptococci (*Streptococcus pyogenes*) are one of the main causes of local or systemic infection. The more common mechanism of spread is likely to be through respiratory droplets or the skin, and they may cause a range of infections, including pharyngitis, impetigo, rheumatic fever and glomerulonephritis.
- Group B streptococci (*Streptococcus agalactiae*) are associated with the female genital tract, and are an important cause of neonatal sepsis and meningitis. In some countries screening for Group B streptococci is undertaken as an antenatal procedure in order that the mothers can be treated prophylactically prior to giving birth.
- *Enterococcus faecalis* is part of the normal enteric flora and may cause urinary tract infections, endocarditis and, in immunocompromised patients, severe septicaemia after surgery.
- *Streptococcus pneumoniae* are commensals of the upper respiratory tract, and can cause pneumonia, sinusitis, bacteraemia and meningitis.

Gram-negative cocci

Gram-negative cocci are not a significant cause of healthcare-associated infections, although two important pathogens are *Neisseria gonorrhoeae* and *N. meningitidis* which appear as Gram-negative diplococci (that individually or in pairs may appear as kidney-shaped organisms), the former being associated with the genito-urinary tract (causing the sexually transmitted infection, gonorrhoea), and the latter with the respiratory tract, potentially causing meningococcal meningitis (Brooks et al 2001).

Gram-negative rods (Enterobacteriaceae)

The enterobacteriaceae are an important group of bacteria, in that they are a large group of organisms that inhabit the intestinal tract of humans and animals, with a potential to cause disease (Brooks et al 2001). Some are natural commensals of the human gut, e.g. *Escherichia coli,* that will cause infection opportunistically, whereas others, e.g. *Shigella, Salmonella*, are pathogenetic to humans. They are either facultative anaerobes or aerobes, are motile, have a complex range of antigens and produce a range of toxins. The two main infections in the category are *Escherichia coli* and *Klebsiella pneumoniae.*

- *Escherichia coli* is part of the normal gut flora, and probably provides a beneficial function within that environment. It tends to cause infections when outside of its normal environment, most notably urinary tract infections, sepsis in immune-incompetent patients and meningitis in infants. Strain 0157 has particularly been identified as the cause of haemolytic-uraemic syndrome in children through the expression of a verotoxin, with the bacterium being ingested in undercooked food, or faecal–oral contamination following contact with farm animals (poor hand hygiene).
- *Klebsiella pneumoniae* is carried in the respiratory and alimentary tract of a proportion of normal people. Under normal circumstances it does not cause problems, but can cause pneumonia or urinary tract infections in compromised patients.

Other bacterial infections to note are Salmonellae, Clostridia, Pseudomonads, Acinetobacters and Mycobacteria.

Salmonellae

Salmonellae are a wide range of organisms that are potentially pathogenic to humans. They occur within animal populations and are transferred through the faecal–oral route by ingestion of contaminated foodstuffs and other materials (Brooks et al 2001). Salmonellae are primarily classified into three main groups, with multiple sub-types:

- The enteric (typhoid) fevers. The principal organism in this group is *S. typhi* and, following ingestion of contaminated foodstuffs, the bacterium is absorbed through the small intestine, causing severe systemic illness. Prior to the introduction of antibiotics, *S. typhi* was associated with significant mortality.

- Bacteraemia with focal lesions. This can be caused by ingestion of any of the salmonella strains. Whilst causing significant systemic infection through the blood stream to the focal area, it does not normally present with intestinal symptomology. Treatment is with antimicrobial agents.
- Enterocolitis. This is the most common presentation occurring from any of the 2000 identified sub-species. In this presentation antibiotic treatment is not usually required and may extend the course of infection; treatment is normally restricted to management of symptoms and rehydration where necessary. Globally commonly occurring from any source where food and liquids may become contaminated with faeces from infected animals, poultry or shellfish, and from handling of animals that may be carriers, e.g. terrapins.

Clostridia

Clostridia are anaerobic, spore-forming organisms that cause a range of disease in man, primarily through the release of exotoxins (Brooks et al 2001). The clostridia are primarily found within the environment, although *C. difficile* is thought primarily to be a part of the normal human gut flora. Three clostridia infections are discussed here.

- *Clostridium difficile* is primarily a cause of diarrhoeal disease through the release of toxins. The organism may be a normal part of the gut flora (present in approximately 3% of the UK adult population) (Health Protection Agency 2010), and usually causes no disease as it is suppressed by the normal gut flora. However, in the event of changes to the equilibrium of the gut through the administration of broad spectrum antibiotics, gut surgery, or changes in the immune status of the patient, the organism can proliferate and cause significant infection. Symptomatic patients may cause environmental contamination with the organism, which persists/survives for extended periods of time as spores that resist drying, and may be ingested by other patients causing outbreaks of infection. The organism releases cytopathic toxins and enterotoxins that cause a range of disease from self-limiting diarrhoea to pseudomembranous colitis and toxic mega colon, which, if untreated, may be fatal. Treatment is initially with antibiotics, but in severe cases may require radical surgery in the form of colectomy as a life-saving intervention.

- *Clostridium perfringens* is found in the environment. It enters the body through trauma (or can be related to gut surgery) and is primarily a cause of gas gangrene through the production of toxins. The toxins are necrotising haemolytic alpha toxins, which cause tissue necrosis and haemolysis potentiating the effectiveness of the anaerobic bacteria by providing a suitable environment. *C. perfringens* is also a recognised cause of toxin-induced food poisoning.
- *Clostridium tetani* is found in the environment and causes tetanus. Tetanus is preventable and is part of national vaccination programmes in many countries. *C. tetani* usually gains entrance to the body through environmental contamination of dirty wounds. Infection is not dependant on the degree of trauma, and may be associated with relatively minor wounds.

Pseudomonads and acinetobacters

- *Pseudomonas* spp. These are important pathogens, particularly in hospitalised, immunocompromised patients (Brooks et al 2001). Pseudomonads occur widely in soil and water, and thus in plants and animals, and are capable of colonising the hospital environment, with subsequent risk of infection to susceptible patients. *Pseudomonas aeruginosa* is the main pathogen of this group, and in situations where it can become established in a patient will excrete exotoxins that may cause tissue necrosis and may be of sufficient severity to be lethal to the individual. It may invade wounds, the respiratory tract, the urinary tract and the blood stream, resulting in fatal sepsis.
- *Acinetobacter* spp. These are not significant pathogens, however, being widely present in the environment in water and the soil, are associated with infections in immunocompromised patients, colonising the respiratory tract via contaminated humidifiers, or as an opportunistic infection of burns and wounds in these patients. Acinetobacters have a level of resistance to antimicrobial agents and are of concern in that they may be difficult to treat and eradicate.

Mycobacteria

The mycobacteria are rod-shaped aerobic bacteria that do not form spores (Brooks et al 2001). Due to their 'waxy' cell wall they do not readily stain, although once stained they are resistant to decolourisation and are referred to as acid-fast bacilli. The process of staining is known as the Ziehl-Neelsen technique. Two mycobacteria are *M. tuberculosis* and *M. kansasii.*

• *M. tuberculosis* (Tb) is a cause of significant infection globally in man (*M. bovis* in cattle) which, untreated, has a significant morbidity and mortality, especially in populations where malnutrition and deprivation are rife. Successful treatment of Tb is primarily with combination antimicrobial therapy, normally with three drugs, for an extended period. Combination therapy is given to reduce the risk of drug resistance occurring. Tb causes both primary and secondary (reactivation) infection. Primary infection is as a consequence of the initial inoculation with the bacterium causing an acute inflammatory response at the site of infection, usually in the lung bases. Tubercle bacilli are spread by both the lymphatic system and the blood stream; distribution by the blood stream may result in the infection of other organs and is known as miliary Tb.
• *M. kansasii* may cause systemic and respiratory disease, particularly affecting severely immunocompromised patients, and is specifically associated with patients with advanced human immunodeficiency virus (HIV) infection.

Key points

• Most bacterial infections are opportunist, in that they occur when the body's immune system is compromised
• Although antimicrobial resistance may occur, timely treatment with appropriate antimicrobial agents will normally be effective
• The effect of infection will be dependent on the type of organism, e.g. enzyme or toxin producers will have differing modes of action
• In some infections, surgical intervention is essential to limit the degree of damage, e.g. necrotising fasciitis

---

Other infections

Whilst we have placed particular emphasis on bacterial infections, it is important to note other non-bacterial infections that might be encountered within the healthcare environment. These include those caused by fungi, protozoa, and viruses.

Viruses

Most viral infections are relatively short-lived and are self-limiting, e.g. influenza, with some conferring immunity to the host, e.g. measles, varicella. However, others may cause more significant infection, e.g. human immunodeficiency virus (HIV), Hepatitis B virus and Hepatitis C virus.

Fungi

Few fungi cause significant disease in man except in immunocompromised patients. They are divided into those that cause superficial infections, such as ringworm (*Tinea corporis*) or athletes' foot (*Tinea pedis*), and those that may cause deep infection (*Aspergillus fumigates*).

Protozoa

Protozoa are known to cause a range of disease in man, most notably malaria (*Plasmodium*), amoebic dysentery (*Entamoeba histolytica*), or other diarrhoeal disease (*Cryptosporidia* spp.).

Chain of infection

Effective infection prevention and control is achieved through an understanding of the infective organism's disease processes, its requirements, how it is transmitted and how it gains entrance to the body to cause infection. This understanding enables effective interventions that break that process. This is often portrayed as a cycle known as the chain of infection. The number of links within the chain is debatable, but it usually consists of six links, as portrayed in *Figure 2.4*. The principles of the chain of infection can be applied within any healthcare setting. These principles are also applicable in the food industry, animal husbandry, water and sanitation processes, etc.

I. Infectious agent – bacterium, virus, fungus, etc.

For an infection to take place there has to be an infectious agent. Not all organisms

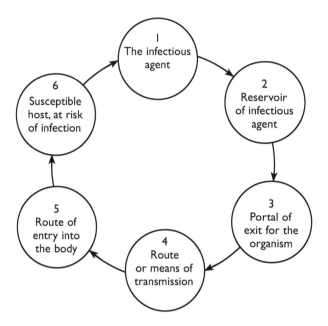

Figure 2.4. The chain of infection.

present the same level of pathogenicity, and will require both sufficient numbers and time to cause an infection; an ability to overcome the host's immune response; an ability to create or adapt to a suitable environment; and adequate nutrients to enable growth to occur.

2. Reservoir of infection

The reservoir is where the organism may survive, e.g. in people, animals, food, water, the environment, etc. The organisms can be eliminated through protection of susceptible individuals by isolation of infectious patients, immunisation programmes, testing for humans and animals, good food hygiene and management, proactive water management programmes, etc.

3. Portal of exit

The portal of exit is where the infection can be transmitted from its reservoir, e.g. via skin, droplets, secretions, excreta, etc.

4. Route of transmission

This refers to accessing the susceptible host, e.g. contact, inhalation, ingestion, injection, etc. When considering where effective interventions are best placed in infection prevention and control, interruption of transmission is a key point for action. Fundamental to breaking the chain is the prevention of direct contact through effective hand hygiene and the proper use of personal protective equipment. The risk of infection by injection can be minimised by safe sharps practice, although different strategies are required when considering insect-borne infections, such as malaria.

5. Route of entry

This how the organism gains entry to the body, e.g. through wounds, urinary tract, alimentary canal, respiratory tract, etc. When considering the routes of entry they should be divided into two groups: those that normally exist, e.g. mouth and nose, and those that are created through instrumentation. In the latter group, when considering a patient's risk of infection it is essential that best practice measures are adopted to protect the patient, primarily through the appropriate use of aseptic technique. Aseptic non-touch technique has been described by Rowley (2001) and is a recognised programme for minimising the risk of introduction of pathogenic bacteria during and after instrumentation of patients.

6. Susceptible host

A susceptible host is any individual or population at risk of infection, e.g. immunocompromised patients, through instrumentation, damaged skin, or chemotherapy, or in those without immunity to specific infections. At risk patients or other individuals can be protected effectively through immunisation programmes, protective and source isolation from and to infectious individuals, the adoption of programmes such as the aseptic non-touch technique, prophylactic antimicrobial therapy, etc. Most important of all is effective hand hygiene between patient contacts.

Summary

This chapter has looked at various types of microorganisms that cause diseases in patients. It has examined the classification of these organisms, given examples of microorganisms of note, and detailed the specific types of infections that can result. The various stages of the growth cycle of microorganisms have been highlighted and specifically the chain of infection to demonstrate the cycle necessary for an infection to occur. However, this chapter can be no more than an overview of the key characteristics of microorganisms, and as such more detailed reading is strongly recommended to fully understand their complexities and the mechanisms by which they grow, survive and, in some cases, cause disease. A brief list of suggested further reading is supplied below. This wider understanding is essential in attempting to apply effective infection prevention and control.

In the next chapter we will look specifically at how the transmission of these microorganisms occurs and the effects they can cause in an otherwise healthy individual.

References

Brooks GF, Butel JS, Morse SA (2001) *Jawetz, Melnick and Adelberg's Medical Microbiology* (22nd edn). Prentice-Hall International, Conneticut USA

Health Protection Agency (2010).Available from: http://www.hpa.org.uk/infections/topics_az/clostridium_difficile/default.htm

Hempel S (2007) *The medical detective – John Snow, cholera and the mystery of the Broad Street pump*. Granta Books, London

McInnes EM (1990) *St Thomas' Hospital* (2nd edn). St Thomas' Hospital, London

Mims C, Playfair J, Roitt I, Wakelin D, Williams R (1998) *Medical microbiology* (2nd edn). Moseby, London

Nightingale F (1860) *Notes on Nursing – What it is and what it is not*. Dover Publications, New York, USA

Rowley S (2001) Aseptic non-touch technique. *Nursing Times Plus* 97(7): vi–viii

Wilson J (2006) *Infection control in clinical practice* (3rd edn). Bailliere Tindall, London

Further reading

Brooks GF, Butel JS, Morse SA (2001) *Jawetz, Melnick and Adelberg's Medical Microbiology* (22nd edn). Prentice-Hall International, Conneticut USA

Perry C (2007) *Infection prevention and control*. Blackwell Publishing, Oxford

Wilson J (2006) *Infection control in clinical practice* (3rd edn). Bailliere Tindall, London

CHAPTER 3

Means of transmission of infectious agents

Sheila Loveridge

Purpose

The purpose of this chapter is to provide an overview of how infectious agents are transmitted across a variety of healthcare settings and individuals. It looks specifically at the use of invasive medical devices and how infections can be introduced through these means.

Learning outcomes

By the end of the chapter, you will have learned:

- The common activities of pathogens.
- Direct and indirect contact transmission.
- The main classes of parasites.
- The role of the skin in protection from infection.
- Transmission through invasive medical devices.

Introduction

In the mid-19th century, the popular hypothesis behind disease transmission was the miasma theory. This theory, which held that disease was transmitted through a poisonous mist or vapours containing particles of decomposed matter and accompanied by a foul smell, was supported by Florence Nightingale. It was thought that the miasma could be eliminated by thorough cleaning and the ensuring of good ventilation. Even though the miasma theory was disproved, the connection between dirt and diseases was made. The miasma theory understood that disease was associated with poor sanitation and that sanitary improvements reduced disease.

For a disease to be caused, pathogens must be able to enter the body of the host, adhering to specific cells within the host, in addition to colonising, infecting and damaging tissues. A pathogen is an agent that causes disease, such as bacteria or viruses.

Activities of pathogens

Entry into the body of the host can typically occur through the mouth, eyes or genital openings, or through wounds that breach the skin barrier to pathogens. Even though some pathogens can grow at the original entry site, to cause an infection most must invade areas of the body where they are not normally found. This is done by the pathogen attaching itself to specific host cells. Some pathogens then reproduce between host cells or within body fluids, while others, such as viruses and some bacterial species, enter the host cells and grow there.

In some cases, the growth of pathogens may be enough to cause tissue damage. In others, however, damage is usually inflicted by the production of toxins or destructive enzymes by the pathogen. An example of this is the bacterium *Streptococcus pyogenes*. This bacterium can cause several types of infection such as pharyngitis (strep throat), impetigo or cellulitis. However, it also can produce enzymes that break down barriers between epithelial cells and remove fibrin clots, helping the bacteria invade tissues and resulting in necrotising fasciitis, a much more serious condition.

Box 3.1 shows the five main routes through which microorganisms are transmitted. In terms of nosocomial or healthcare-associated infections, the first three routes are of major importance.

Transmission of infection requires at least three elements: a source of infecting microorganisms, a susceptible host and a means of transmission for bacteria and viruses. *Figure 3.1* illustrates these three elements.

The environment is full of microorganisms, many of which do not cause harm. However, pathogenic microorganisms also exist, and these can be easily spread, especially in healthcare environments. In the mid-1800s, Ignaz Semmelweis made

---

Box 3.1. Five main routes for the transmission of microorganisms

- Direct contact
- Droplets
- Airborne
- Common vehicle
- Vector borne

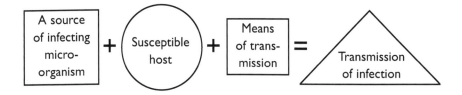

Figure 3.1. Elements for transmission of infection.

the first connection regarding the transfer of pathogenic bacteria from healthcare worker to patient. In introducing hand washing in between patients, he reduced the rates of puerperal sepsis in childbirth amongst women in the hospital and began the basis of infection control practice.

Contact transmission

Direct

There are two methods of contact transmission of infectious agents: direct or indirect. Direct contact occurs when an individual is infected by contact with the reservoir where the infectious agent is found. This normally consists of person-to-person contact and physical transfer of microorganisms between a susceptible host and a colonised or infected individual. Infectious agents, for example gonorrhoea (*Neisseria gonorrhoeae*) can be contracted through intimate sexual contact in this manner. Contact of an uninfected person with infected wounds or blood may result in direct transmission of viruses, such as the human immunodeficiency virus (HIV). Needlestick injuries are a possible source of transmission of blood-borne viruses.

Indirect

Indirect contact occurs when a pathogen can survive in the environment outside its host for a long period of time before infecting another individual. Inanimate objects, such as medical instruments, or equipment used in food preparation that are contaminated by direct contact with the reservoir could be the indirect contact for a susceptible individual, and in turn spread the disease to other individuals. Food-borne illnesses occur when food contaminated with microorganisms is ingested. Infected needles may be the source of indirect transmission of pathogens between intravenous drug users. Healthcare workers' hands may also cause the transmission of infectious particles from patient to patient if adequate hand washing practices are not rigorously followed. This mode of transmission on hands is a common cause of healthcare-associated infections.

Ingestion

As mentioned above, ingesting food and beverages contaminated by contact with a disease reservoir is another example of transmission by indirect contact. The faecal–oral route of transmission, in which sewage-contaminated water is used for drinking, washing, or preparing foods, is a significant form of indirect transmission, especially for gastrointestinal diseases such as cholera. This is also known by the term 'common vehicle spread'. This describes the mode of transmission of infectious pathogens from a source that is common to all the cases of a specific disease, by means of a medium, or 'vehicle', such as water, food, air or other factors, e.g. blood transfusion. Transmission by the faecal–oral route is the second most significant mode of transmission after the respiratory tract.

Droplet transmission

Droplet transmission occurs when infectious droplets are generated during coughing, sneezing or talking or through medical procedures such as suctioning. These droplets can be propelled several metres through the air and deposited on a host's mouth, nasal mucosa or conjunctivae, or can be inhaled. The droplets are generally 10 micrometers or greater in size. Droplet transmission is not to be confused with airborne transmission because droplets do not remain suspended in the air or travel in air currents and special air handling and ventilation is not required. Droplet transmission is also considered to be a direct transmission of pathogens. An example of a virus spread by droplet transmission is influenza.

Dental route

Dental water supplies have been implicated as a vehicle for the transmission of microorganisms. Biofilms form rapidly on dental unit waterlines. The majority of the organisms in the biofilm are harmless environmental species, but some dental units may harbour opportunistic respiratory pathogens. Jensen et al (1997) investigated the presence of *Pseudomonas aeruginosa* in dental water supplies and the possible link to positive sputum in cystic fibrosis patients.

Airborne

Airborne transmission occurs when dust particles containing bacteria or airborne droplets become aerosolised and remain suspended in the air for longer durations of time. The particles are generally five micrometres or less in diameter. Small droplet nuclei and aerosols can remain suspended in the air for prolonged periods and can travel significant distances. Small particles are thought to be more infectious, with both the degree of infectivity and the severity of illness directly related to particle size. Microorganisms transmitted in this manner can be inhaled by a susceptible host, so special air handling is indicated to prevent the spread of infection. An example of a bacterium spread by airborne transmission is *Mycobacterium tuberculosis*.

Common vehicle

Blood and blood products

Throughout the 1970s and the first half of the 1980s, many haemophiliacs and other patients in the UK were treated with blood and blood products that carried Hepatitis C, and some 4670 patients became infected. Between 1983 and the early 1990s some 1200 patients were infected with HIV, also through blood products

---

Case study: Common vehicle spread

A historical example of common vehicle spread was the water pump in Broad Street, Soho, which was the source of the cholera outbreak in London, August 1854. During this time, it was assumed that cholera was spread by airborne transmission, using the miasma theory. However, John Snow did not accept this, and argued that the disease entered the body through the mouth. Snow published his theories (1855) and was able to prove one in somewhat dramatic circumstances.

In August 1854, a cholera outbreak occurred in Soho. After careful investigation, including plotting cases of cholera on a map of the area, Snow was able to identify a water pump in Broad (now Broadwick) Street as the source of the disease. He had the handle of the pump removed, and cases of cholera immediately began to diminish. However, Snow's 'germ' theory of disease was not widely accepted until the 1860s.

(Archer et al 2009). Transmission of HIV by transfusion has become increasingly rare in developed countries since the commencement of screening of donors at risk for HIV infection, and routine HIV antibody testing of all donations. Continued improvement in donor recruitment practices, donor education, donor screening, and blood testing has resulted in continued decreases in the risk of transfusion transmission of HIV (Donegan et al 1994).

However, the risk of HIV transfusion through infected blood products remains greater than any other risk exposure. Ninety percent of recipients who have received a transfusion with HIV antibody-positive blood are found to be HIV infected at follow-up (Donegan et al 1994). Globally, the risk of contracting HIV through contaminated blood products is much higher. HIV infection transmitted through transfusion is thought to account for 80000–160000 infections annually, contributing 2–4% of all cases of HIV transmission (Noel 2002, Goodnough et al 2003).

Funding considerations play a major part in this issue and lead to outcomes such as inadequate HIV testing. However this is only part of the problem. Specific issues that need to be addressed urgently include the lack of a sufficient volunteer blood donor pool in underdeveloped countries, and inadequate blood donor screening, information, counselling, and confidentiality. In many countries, to be identified as HIV positive carries an enormous social stigma. In some areas of Kenya, for example, men send their wives for HIV testing to determine their own status, rather than be tested themselves. HIV positive women are subsequently abandoned and ostracised.

Education is the most important component of a screening programme, which should also include implementation of standardised and monitored test manufacturing practices, inclusion of test validation procedures, ongoing staff training, and continuous internal and external quality assessment programmes. All these are necessary to provide an effective programme to prevent transmission. Transfusion practices should be monitored locally to reduce the risk of HIV transmission from unnecessary transfusions.

Artificial insemination

Another means of transmission of infectious agents, albeit low risk, is through sperm. Women known to be infected with HIV through receiving infected sperm are mainly those who were inseminated before the availability of HIV antibody testing. Sperm washing (a process where centrifugation, repeated washing, and an incubation period that allows spermatozoa to swim to the upper layer of the culture medium is carried out) is a practice used successfully by several centres in Europe (Mayer 1999). Although this procedure involves some risk of HIV transmission, it may offer reduced risk for couples seeking artificial insemination, where one or both partners are HIV positive.

Vector-borne infection

Vector-borne infection occurs through transmission of a pathogen via an animal or insect into a human host. Transmission in this manner requires three different living organisms: the pathogen, the vector and the human host. An example of this is the malarial parasite which is transmitted to the host through the bite of an infected mosquito. Lyme disease is another well-known bacterial infection, the source of which is the microorganism *Borrelia burgdorferi,* which is transmitted to humans by the bite of infected blacklegged ticks.

***

Key points

Infection can be transmitted through the following routes:
- Direct contact
- Droplets
- Dental water
- Airborne
- Ingestion
- Blood and blood products
- Artificial insemination of sperm
- Vector borne

***

Parasites

Parasitic microorganisms live on or in a host organism and obtain their nutrients from or at the expense of their host. There are three main classes of parasites that can cause disease in humans. These are:

- Protozoa.
- Giardia.
- Helminths.

Protozoa

Protozoa are single-celled, microscopic organisms that can perform all the necessary functions of metabolism and reproduction. Some protozoa are free-living, but others act as parasites in other organisms to enable them to acquire their nutrients and continue their life cycle. An example is *Cryptosporidium* spp. These are gastrointestinal parasites that are spread through the faecal–oral route. Many species of *Cryptosporidium* exist that infect both humans and animals. The parasite is protected by an outer shell that allows it to survive outside the body for long periods of time and makes it extremely resistant to chlorine disinfection. While this parasite can be spread in several different ways, water is a common method of transmission and *Cryptosporidium* is one of the most frequent causes of water-borne disease.

Giardia

Giardiasis is another disease caused by a microscopic parasite, *Giardia intestinalis* (also known as *Giardia lamblia* or *Giardia duodenalis*). Again, this organism is spread through the faecal–oral route. Once a person or animal has been infected, the parasite continues to live in the intestine and is passed in faeces. Because the parasite is protected by an outer shell, it can survive outside the body and in the environment for long periods of time. *Toxoplasma* (*Toxoplasma gondii*) and *Trichomonas* (*Trichomonas vaginalis*) are further examples of protozoal microorganisms that cause disease.

Helminths

Helminths are large, multicellular organisms that are generally visible to the naked eye in the adult stage. Helminths can be free-living or parasitic. An example

---

Key points

- Parasites are organisms that live on or in other organisms from which they obtain nutrients to live. They can cause harm in the process
- Parasitic diseases in humans are caused by protozoans and helminths
- Most parasites require a host to complete their life cycle
- Ectoparasites are those that live on skin or attach to hair follicles

---

of a disease caused by this type of microorganism is schistosomiasis, also known as bilharzia. This is a disease caused by parasitic worms, such as *Schistosoma mansoni, Schistosoma haematobium* and *Schistosoma japonicum*. The infection occurs when human skin comes in contact with contaminated freshwater in which certain types of snails that carry schistosomes are living. More than 200 million people are infected worldwide, mainly in developing countries.

Ectoparasites

Ectoparasites are a classification of animals that includes those with hard, segmented bodies and jointed appendages, such as insects. Ectoparasites are usually arthropods that live on the skin but do not enter the body of the host. Although the term ectoparasite can include blood-sucking arthropods, e.g. mosquitoes, it is generally used to describe organisms such as ticks, fleas, lice, and mites that attach or burrow into the skin and remain there for relatively long periods of time. Arthropods are important in causing diseases in their own right, but are even more important as vectors of many different microorganisms that cause disease.

Horizontal and vertical modes of transmission

The modes of transmission described above are considered to be horizontal because the infectious agent can be passed from person to person within a group. Vertical transmission, also known as perinatal transmission, occurs when the disease is transmitted from parent to child in utero during fetal development, through the placenta or, after birth, through breastfeeding. In some cases it is difficult to differentiate between perinatal or transplacental transmission, since both are known to occur.

An example of vertical transmission of disease is when an infant contracts early onset Group B *Streptococcus* infection during vaginal birth. Gonorrhoea (*Neisseria gonorrhoeae*), syphilis (*Treponema pallidum*) and chlamydia (*Chlamydia trachomatis*) are also examples of microorganisms that can be spread by vertical transmission, resulting in infection in the newborn as well as the mother. Even a seemingly innocuous infection, such as dental caries, can be transmitted from mother to child. *Streptococcus mutans* and *Streptococcus sobrinus* are known to be the most prevalent caries-associated organisms in humans. The mother–child infection route of *Streptococcus mutans* can be prevented by simply reducing the amount of microorganisms contained in the mothers' saliva (Hanada 2000).

A healthy intact skin is one of the greatest defences from infection, since microorganisms are unable to pierce unbroken skin. When the skin is broken, either intentionally or unintentionally, the risk of microorganisms entering the body system is increased. Ayton (1985) defines the loss of continuity of skin or tissue as a wound, which may result from accidental trauma, an underlying disease process or a surgical procedure.

Infection via the skin

Surgical wounds

Surgical wound infections account for between 10% and 20% of infections acquired in hospital (Emmerson et al 1996). During the procedure, microorganisms may be introduced into the incision and, depending on the type of surgery, can result in infection, either superficial, deep, in organs or at other sites, such as joints. The bacteria may be introduced from a variety of sources but the most common is the patients' own microbial flora (Wilson 2006). The balance between the strength of the host's immune system and the number of pathogenic bacteria in the wound will influence the risk of infection. The number of bacteria will be dependant on the operation site. Bowel surgery, for example, may carry a higher risk of infection.

Burns

Burns carry a high risk of infection through colonising microorganisms. Weber et al (1997) state that patients with burns on 60% or more of their body are most vulnerable, with two thirds developing infection on the burns themselves, and most developing a secondary bloodstream infection. The risk of transmission of microorganisms on burn units is high, with the main factors being contaminated hands or equipment. The large surface area of damaged skin increases the probability of microorganisms being introduced from an airborne route, particularly those bacteria that are more resistant to desiccation, such as *Staphylococcus* and *Acinetobacter* (Wilson 1996).

Chronic wounds

Chronic wounds such as ulcers and pressure sores, as well as non-healing burns and surgical wounds, are often a reservoir of microorganisms from the surrounding skin, all of which can be easily transmitted. Bloodstream infections originating from chronic wounds are becoming more common and healing these wounds is the most effective way of reducing transmission. However, successful healing may often depend on underlying problems and may be impaired by issues such as poor blood supply.

Activity

- Within your clinical area, consider patients who have the following:
  - A surgical wound after an operation
  - A chronic wound such as a pressure ulcer
  - Burns after a scalding accident
- What actions will you take to minimise the risk of infection to the patient, to the visitor, and to yourself?
- How would you care for this patient?

Infections via invasive devices

Intravenous catheters

Another method of transmission of microorganisms is through invasive devices. Glynn et al's (1997) surveillance study found that over 60% of patients admitted to hospital will receive therapy via an intravenous (IV) catheter. Bloodstream infections, although not common, can occur when microorganisms colonising the skin and surface of the invasive device are released into the bloodstream, where they can easily multiply and cause infection. Secondary infections can also be caused by bacteria attaching to other tissues in the body. Examples of this, given by Haase et al (2005), are osteomyelitis, endocarditis and endophthalmitis.

There are a variety of intravenous devices. These range from cannulae, which are inserted peripherally, to central lines, inserted into the chest. There are a host of central venous access devices used for a variety of purposes, such as the giving of antibiotics and chemotherapy. Peripherally inserted central catheters (PICC) are inserted into one of the cephalic, basilic or median cubital veins in an adult arm and used to deliver chemotherapy or antibiotics. Midlines are placed just above or below the fold of the antecubital area, or higher up the arm with ultrasound use. Midline catheters are used where patients present with poor peripheral venous access and when the use of a central venous catheter is contraindicated (Griffiths 2007). Short-term central venous catheters, Hickman lines, skin-tunnelled catheters and implanted ports are other examples of intravenous devices that can transmit microorganisms if not handled correctly and aseptically.

Hickman lines and totally implanted or subcutaneous central venous systems carry the lowest risk of infection. The former has an estimated incidence of infection at 1.4 per 1000 catheter days, compared to 3 per 1000 catheter days with non-tunnelled central vascular catheters (Widner 1997). Subcutaneous central venous systems such as the Port-a-Cath have an estimated risk of 0.2 infections per 1000 catheter days (Groeger et al 1993).

Bacteria colonising the skin site can gain access to the blood vessel by migrating along the outside of the intravenous catheter. A strong association is often seen between the culture of microorganisms from the insertion site and those grown from a catheter tip after removal. Contamination of the catheter hub results in bacteria travelling through the catheter lumen, protected from the host immune system defences and colonising the catheter tip. Manipulation of intravenous devices is known to add to the risk of infection.

Parenteral nutrition feeding is another source of transmission. The administration of nutrients into a vein via a central venous catheter gives rise to a possibility of contamination. The parenteral nutrition fluid is an ideal medium in which bacteria will multiply. Proper insertion and care of catheters is essential to avoid infection.

The percentage of catheter-related infections is lower for single-lumen than for multi-lumen catheters. Farkas et al (1992) reported a large difference: 11.5% for single-lumen versus 16.2% for multi-lumen. Although the reason for the decreased risk of infection associated with use of single-lumen catheters remains unproved, it was felt to be most likely due to less manipulation. Multi-lumen catheters can be used to administer multiple medications during multiple intervals. Therefore these catheters are manipulated many more times than single-lumen catheters. The chance of a break in the sterile barrier and resultant infection is higher for the multi-lumen devices.

Another possible cause of transmission of microorganisms is through contaminated infusate or multi-use vials. In many cases, a short-sighted desire to save money results in the contents of large vials being used multiple times and accessed inappropriately. There are many examples where this practice has led to contamination in multi-dose vials and therefore this practice should not be encouraged, to reduce the risk of transmission. Contaminated ophthalmic solutions can also represent a potential cause of avoidable ocular infection

---

Activity

Mr Peters has returned to your ward following a surgical procedure. He has in place two intravenous lines and parenteral nutrition feeding has been commenced through an intravascular line. The doctor has prescribed intravenous medication to be given four times a day.
• What are the risks of transmission of infection via these routes?
• How would you minimise these?

(Nentwich et al 2007). Single dose vials should not be reused and, as with any infusate or medication, strict aseptic techniques are essential during handling to prevent extrinsic contamination and dangerous complications from infection.

Urinary catheters

Urinary tract infections (UTIs) are estimated by Emmerson et al (1996) to account for over 20% of healthcare-associated infections. Plowman et al (2001) estimated that approximately 2.5% of patients admitted to hospital had or would acquire a urinary tract infection, with associated increased costs and length of stay. A prospective case control study by Nguyen-Van-Tam et al (1999) identified female sex, increased length of stay, elective admission, surgical operation, and transurethral and repeated intermittent catheterisation as significant independent risk factors for hospital-acquired urinary tract infection (HAUTI). However, specialty of admission was also a significant risk factor when added to the model and, under these conditions, only length of stay and catheterisation remained significant.

Under normal circumstances, the bladder has several defences against the transmission of microorganisms. In the lining of the bladder itself, there are epithelial cells that are resistant to bacterial attachment. The urethra is generally difficult for microorganisms to enter and pass along. Urination ensures that any bacteria that manage to enter the urethra do not gain access to the bladder itself; they are diluted and flushed out of the body by the flow of urine. The insertion of a urinary catheter bypasses these defences and predisposes the patient to developing a urinary tract infection. Elderly and debilitated patients and others who are catheterised for long periods of time are therefore at greater risk of recurrent urinary tract infections and developing long-term complications, including urinary sepsis.

The microorganisms that commonly cause urinary tract infections are those, such as *Escherichia coli,* which can be found colonising the periurethral area. In a non-catheterised patient, *E coli* can cause serious infections and tissue damage. The need for cleanliness and good hygiene is paramount to avoid infection. In catheterised patients, there is a greater variety of microorganisms that can cause a catheter-associated urinary tract infection (CAUTI). Yeasts are a frequent example of microorganisms found in CAUTIs. Catheters that are in place for a long time show a greater variety of bacteria identified in the urine during culture.

There are three ways in which microorganisms can enter the body. Firstly, contamination may occur if there has been a poor mechanical insertion procedure or the correct aseptic technique was not followed during the insertion stage; either of these may allow the introduction of bacteria. Secondly, as with an intravenous device, bacteria may travel along the outside of a catheter. This may happen as the catheter is inserted, either from the healthcare workers' hands or the patient's own perianal flora. Finally, bacteria may be able to travel along the inside lumen of a catheter. This is usually through reflux of urine from a contaminated catheter bag.

There are differences in these routes of infection, depending on whether the patient is male or female. Due to the perineum's placement on the body, it is frequently colonised by bacteria which normally are found in the gut. In a female, the urethra is relatively short and therefore it is easier for bacteria from the perineum to reach the bladder. Genital and perianal cleansing is therefore a very important part of daily hygiene. The presence of a catheter probably accounts for a significant proportion of urinary tract infections in catheterised women (Daifuku and Stamm 1984).

In men, the urethra is longer and further away from the rectum, thereby reducing the risk of contamination. Research has shown that the most common cause of urinary tract infection in catheterised men is through cross-infection via the lumen of the catheter, possibly due to the handling of the urine system when it is emptied, disconnected or otherwise handled (Daifuku and Stamm 1984).

Residual urine in the bladder of catheterised patients increases the risk of urinary tract infection. During the process of infection, bacteria need first to adhere to the epithelial cells of the urinary tract and/or surface of the catheter. They will then develop into biofilms on the catheter surface and are resistant to the immune system and antibiotics. Catheters by themselves may cause immediate physical damage to the bladder epithelium; they may be toxic and also cause inflammation (Barford and Coates 2009). The Cochrane Review of silver alloy-coated Foley catheters concluded that they are successful at reducing the rate of this healthcare-associated infection, which can be potentially fatal (Brosnahan et al 2004).

Antimicrobial coated urinary catheters are also available but possible benefits of antibiotic prophylaxis must be balanced against possible adverse effects, such as development of antibiotic resistant bacteria; these cannot be reliably estimated from currently available trials (Niël-Weise and van den Broek 2005).

Summary

This chapter has looked at the how infectious agents can be transmitted from one individual to another, and some of the main activities of pathogens and parasites. The role of the skin in protection against infection was discussed, and how best practice around the use of invasive medical devices can further reduce patients' exposure to infections. In the next chapter we will look at the role of staff health and immunisation in protecting both patients, visitors and staff from infectious agents.

Key points

To minimise the risk of infection via the urinary catheter the following must be observed:
- Safe procedure during insertion
- Thorough genital and perianal cleaning
- Avoidance of prolonged use of urinary catheters
- Avoidance of residual urine in the bladder of catheterised patients
- Prevention of the reflux of urine from the drainage bag

References

Archer Rt Hon Lord, Jones N, Willetts J (2009) *The Archer Inquiry*. Available from: http://www.archercbbp.com/ [Accessed 5 April 2010]

Ayton M (1985) Wounds that won't heal. *Nursing Times* **81**(46): 16–19

Barford JMT, Coates ARM (2009) The pathogenesis of catheter-associated urinary tract infection. *Journal of Infection Prevention* **10**(2): 50–6

Brosnahan J et al (2004) Types of urethral catheters for management of short-term voiding problems in hospitalised adults (Cochrane Review). *The Cochrane Library*; (Issue 1). Chichester: Wiley

Daifuku R, Stamm W (1984) Association of rectal and urethral colonization with urinary tract infection in patients with indwelling catheters. *Journal of the American Medical*

Association 254: 2028–30

Donegan E, Lee H, Operskalski EA et al (1994) Transfusion transmission of retroviruses: Human T-lymphotropic virus types l and ll compared with human immunodeficiency virus type 1. *Transfusion* **34**: 478–83

Emmerson AM, Enstone JE, Griffin M et al (1996) The second national prevalence study of infection in hospitals – overview of the results. *Journal of Hospital Infection* **32**(3): 175–90

Farkas JC, Liu N, Bleriot JP et al (1992) Single-versus triple-lumen central catheter-related sepsis: A prospective randomised study in a critically ill population. *American Journal of Medicine* **93**: 277–82

Glynn A, Ward V, Wilson J et al (1997) *Hospital acquired infection surveillance policies and practice – study of the control of hospital acquired infection in 19 hospitals in England and Wales.* London: Public Health Laboratory Service

Goodnough LT, Shander A, Brecher ME (2003) Transfusion medicine: Looking to the future. *Lancet* **361**(9352): 161–9

Griffiths V (2007) Midline catheters: Indications, complications and maintenance. *Nursing Standard* **22**(11): 48–57

Groeger JS, Lucas AB, Thaler HT et al (1993) Infectious morbidity associated with long-term use of venous access devices in patients with cancer. *Annals of Internal Medicine* **119**: 1168–74

Haase J, McCracken KA, Akins RL (2005) Catheter-related bloodstream infections in the intensive care unit population. *Journal of Pharmacy Practice* **18**(1): 42–52

Hanada N (2000) Current understanding of the cause of dental caries. *Japanese Journal of Infectious Diseases* **53**(1): 1–5

Jensen ET, Giwercman B, Ojeniyi B, et al (1997) Epidemiology of *Pseudomonas aeruginosa* in cystic fibrosis and the possible role of contamination by dental equipment. *Journal of Hospital Infection* **36**: 117–22

Mayer KH (1999) Risks of human immunodeficiency virus transmission from artificial insemination from an infected donor. *Pediatric Infectious Diseases Journal* **18**(3): 310–1

Nentwich MM, Kollman KHM, Meshack J et al (2007) Microbial contamination of multi-use ophthalmic solutions in Kenya. *British Journal of Ophthalmology* **91**(10): 1265–68

Nguyen-Van-Tam SE, Nguyen-Van-Tam JS, Myint S et al (1999) Risk factors for hospital-acquired urinary tract infection in a large English teaching hospital: A case-control study. *Infection* **27**(3): 192–7

Niël-Weise BS, van den Broek PJ (2005) Urinary catheter policies for long-term bladder drainage. *Cochrane Database of Systematic Reviews*, Issue 1.

Noel L (2002) *Safe blood starts with me, blood saves lives.* Transcripts of World Health Day 2000 Available from: http://www.who.int/multimedia/whd2000/# [Accessed 5 April 2010]

Plowman R, Graves N, Esquive J, Roberts JA (2001) An economic model to assess the cost and benefits of the routine use of silver alloy coated urinary catheters to reduce the risk of urinary tract infections in catheterized patients. *Journal of Hospital Infection* **48**: 38–42

Snow J (1855) *On the mode of communication of cholera*. London: John Churchill. Available from: http://www.ph.ucla.edu/epi/snow/snowbook.html [Accessed 5 April 2010]

Weber JM, Sheridan RL, Pasternack MS et al (1997) Nosocomial infections in paediatric patients with burns. *American Journal of Infection Control* **25**: 145–201

Widner AF (1997) Intravenous-related infections. In Wenzel RP (ed) *Prevention and control of nosocomial infections* (3rd edn). Baltimore: Williams and Wilkins

Wilson J (2006) *Infection control in clinical practice* (3rd edn). London: Bailliere Tindall

Section 2

Prevention and control

CHAPTER 4

Staff health

Dorothy N Chakani

Purpose

This chapter outlines the fundamental aspects of how healthcare workers (HCWs) can protect themselves from occupational infectious diseases. The chapter outlines prevalent risks that HCWs are exposed to in their line of duty and highlights measures required for prudent and safe practice.

Learning outcomes

By the end of the chapter, you will have learned:

*   The role of occupational health in ensuring staff health.
*   Preventative measures for commonly occurring infections, such as respiratory and gastrointestinal infections.
*   Best practice for staying safe and healthy within the healthcare setting.

Introduction

The healthcare environment is full of insidious hazards, the most well known being the risk of patients acquiring healthcare-associated infections (HCAIs). HCWs are also continually at risk of occupationally acquired ill health due to infections, among many other factors.

Studies across the world have shown that HCWs can be severely debilitated by occupationally acquired illness (Puro et al 1995, Avert 2006, Department of Health 2007), which inevitably has a severe impact on healthcare organisations and services. It is imperative that HCWs understand the way infectious diseases occur, how to prevent them and how to protect not only their patients but also themselves.

Several diseases are described in this chapter based on their epidemiological impact and relevance to the HCW. Certain infectious diseases are preventable through vaccinations which enhance the ability of the HCW to resist infections; however other infections have neither vaccines nor absolute treatment. Appropriate and timely exclusion of ill or high risk HCWs and standard infection control precautions are indispensable elements in breaking the chain of infection.

Pre-employment health checks

The occupational health (OH) department is responsible for the health and safety of all healthcare workers employed in the organisation.

Infectious diseases are of concern among HCWs who can serve as highly prolific transmitters of infection. Consequently pre-employment health checks are carried out by prospective employers' OH departments for all new HCWs to ensure their suitability to the job that they have applied for in terms of their health. However, recent recommendations have been made to change this practice and limit pre-employment health checks only to staff applying for jobs where it is deemed essential (Madan and Williams 2010). The pre-employment check assesses the level of risk of the HCW developing work-related illness and also his or her risk of spreading any pre-existing infection. Occupational health personnel are expected to carry out such assessments in an objective and fair manner that is in accordance with good OH practice as well as equal opportunities legislation (NHS Executive 1994).

On completion of the necessary pre-employment health checks OH can thereafter recommend or advise on employment suitability. Healthcare workers considered at risk of exposure to pathogens are offered appropriate pre-exposure immunisations and post-exposure prophylaxis in the unfortunate event of occupational exposure.

Infected HCWs have the same right to confidentiality as any other patient. OH staff work under strict confidentiality guidelines and cannot disclose information about HCWs even to the employer without the individual's consent, except in rare incidents where a patient or the public is or has been put at risk (Department of Health 2007). Should HCWs need to change duties due to an infectious illness, OH will advise the employer of the change and limitations of the change but will not necessarily reveal the diagnosis.

Immunisation

Immunisation is not a substitute for good practice but is an addition to the protection of HCWs (Department of Health 2006). It is essential that all at-risk HCWs, permanent and temporary, are up-to-date with relevant routine immunisations. The status and outcomes of immunisations of HCWs should be obtained and recorded. Although being able to advise on and provide immunisation is a key function of the OH team, the onus is on each HCW to be aware of his or her own current status.

Routine immunisations generally include measles, mumps and rubella (MMR), tetanus, poliomyelitis, and diphtheria. Other vaccines such as Hepatitis B virus (HBV) and Bacille Calmette-Guérin (BCG) are given dependent on the HCW's risk of exposure, for instance HCWs who are at risk of working with tuberculosis (TB) infected patients or possibly in an area where prevalence of patients with TB or suspected TB is high. Hands-on HCWs such as porters, domestic and laundry staff should ideally be vaccinated for HBV. Previous infection of chickenpox is also important to record although no vaccine is available.

Stop, check, ask...

This section has highlighted the importance of ensuring healthcare workers are up to date with their immunisations.
- Are you aware of your current immunisation status for the diseases discussed?
- Have you been exposed to any infections which might place you at risk of disease?
- When was the last time you met with a member from your OH department to discuss your current status?

Staff sickness

The most important resource that any healthcare service has is its staff and staff need to be healthy and fit for work. Staff sickness and absence poses significant staffing and cost implications for healthcare services, and ill health bears a personal financial burden to affected HCWs. In the National Health Service 10.7 million days per year are lost due to HCW sickness and absence, which equates to £1.7 billion per year (Department of Health 2009). The Health and Safety at Work Act (1974) made it a duty for the employer to ensure that working conditions are safe and do not pose a risk to staff health. Similarly HCWs also have a duty to take reasonable care of their own health and safety, as well as that of other people who could be affected due to their acts or omissions at work (Health and Safety at Work Act 1974).

Occupationally acquired infections can result in a range of consequences from inconvenience, to devastation, to fatality, yet a significant proportion of such circumstances are avoidable. Unfortunately, the incidence of occupational infection is under-reported (Health and Safety Executive 2005) and evidence suggests that suboptimal compliance with immunisation and standard infection control precautions are a global phenomenon (Gammon et al 2007, Vagholkar et al 2008).

An example of this phenomenon is that 10–12% of HCWs' sickness and absenteeism globally is attributed to influenza (O'Reilly and Stevens 2002). The socio-economic burden of influenza is unjustifiable as effective vaccinations are generally and freely available to most HCWs, yet uptake remains relatively low. Patients with influenza can easily transmit the infection to unimmunised and susceptible HCWs, who can then be, initially, asymptomatic transmitters of the infection. Sickness and absenteeism is under-reported since, often, HCWs continue to work even when symptomatic due to a multitude of reasons, for instance, poor staffing levels or unpaid sick leave.

Infected HCWs can easily spread infections to susceptible patients and other staff, which can be fatal. A typical renowned example of asymptomatic carriage and spread of infection is that of typhoid Mary, who was a healthy carrier of the typhoid bacteria. Typhoid Mary briefly worked as a cook at a

---

Case study: Typhoid Mary

Mary Mellon worked as a cook for wealthy families in America in the 1900s. She never settled in any of her many jobs as the families she cooked for often became ill. Mary had never been ill and when it was speculated that she was the cause of her employers' illnesses she became very defensive, refusing to cooperate with investigations.

One relentless doctor solicited the help of the police and an ambulance to capture Mary. She was sent to a hospital on a secluded island for a year, where she provided weekly stool specimens and was given treatment.

Mary was eventually released on condition that she signed an affidavit that she would never work as a cook again.

A while after Mary's release she changed her name to Mary Brown and returned to working as a cook, eventually taking up employment at a maternity hospital in New York and there an outbreak of typhoid occurred affecting many patients and staff.

Again she was tracked down and this time returned to the secluded island hospital where she spent the rest of her days.

Wikipedia (2005), Bourdain (2005)

---

women's hospital where she caused a devastating typhoid outbreak (as outlined in the case study).

Exposure to pathogenic microorganisms can cause a multitude of infections which can affect one or multiple areas of the body. The prevalent categories that generally affect HCWs will be discussed in this chapter, namely, gastrointestinal (diarrhoea and vomiting) infections, respiratory infections, blood-borne viral infections and skin infections.

The manner in which pathogens will gain a foothold and cause infections largely depends on an individual's immune response and differing susceptibilities. Consequently symptoms for the same infection may present in various ways. Therefore the symptoms described in this chapter may not be conclusive.

In the next section we will look more closely at some of the most common infections which affect the healthcare worker.

Gastroenteritis

Gastrointestinal infections are amongst the commonest infections in hospitals and the community. Gastroenteritis often presents with diarrhoea and/or vomiting and abdominal pain among other symptoms. Bacteria, viruses or parasites can cause gastrointestinal infection.

Gastroenteritis in the healthcare environment generally spreads through the faecal–oral route either in direct person-to-person contact, or via contaminated food, drink and the environment. There is massive under-reporting of gastrointestinal illness amongst HCWs as they generally 'just endure the illness', often not even staying away from work when ill. Consequently HCWs can become routes of transmission and can spread infection to patients, colleagues, visitors and even their own families. Staff eating and drinking in the clinical environment should be prohibited at all times, as this presents optimal opportunity for exposure to gastrointestinal infections in HCWs.

Key point

The most common causes of gastroenteritis are:
- *Escherichia coli*
- *Salmonella*
- *Campylobacter*
- *Norovirus*

51

HCWs who develop diarrhoea and/or vomiting should stay away from work during their illness for a minimum of 48 hours after their last symptom, to ensure that their symptoms are fully resolved before returning to work. Staying away from work does not warrant taking up extra work elsewhere as this simply increases the sphere of spread of the infection. Faecal specimens should be sent for testing in accordance with local procedures either via the OH department or the HCW's own doctor. One of the most prevalent gastrointestinal infections is *Norovirus,* which accounts for 90% of viral gastroenteritis in humans (Tortora et al 2004). The next section look specifically at *Norovirus.*

Norovirus

Norovirus, also known as the 'winter vomiting disease', accounts for a great deal of discomfort and sickness amongst vulnerable patients and service users within healthcare settings and care homes. This is seen particularly during the winter months. *Norovirus* infection spreads rapidly, although it is self-limiting, and can last 24 to 72 hours. However, the virus can still be excreted in the faeces for up to 10 days after exposure (Chadwick et al 2000).

Incubation and symptoms

Incubation can be up to 48 hours with symptoms of projectile vomiting, profuse diarrhoea, nausea, abdominal cramps, fever and headache.

Prevention

Infected HCWs need to stay away from work during illness with this condition. If working with patients infected with *Norovirus,* the use of personal protective equipment such as aprons and gloves is essential, as well as effective environmental decontamination to prevent further spread. Timely and correct hand washing practice with soap and water is vital. It is important to note that alcohol hand gel is not effective against *Norovirus,* and therefore must not be a substitute for effective hand washing.

Treatment

Although the infection is generally self-limiting, fluid intake should be increased and the HCW should remain at home until 48 hours after symptoms have resolved.

Respiratory infections

Respiratory infections are the most common type of infection, and transmission is via the airborne or droplet route. We will look specifically at two of the main respiratory infections, influenza and *Mycobacterium tuberculosis* (TB).

Influenza (flu)

Influenza is caused by highly infectious *Orthomyxoviridae* viruses that cause acute respiratory tract infection. In healthy people influenza is generally self-limiting within two to seven days. The influenza virus attacks the epithelial cells of the respiratory tract which results in sore throat and can lead to throat and chest infections or pneumonia, often caused by secondary bacterial infection.

There are different types of influenza strains, namely A, B and C. Most clinical illness is caused by A and B types, although it is type A that causes the majority of outbreaks and epidemics (Salisbury et al 2006). The swine flu (H1N1) pandemic of 2009 was a strain of *Influenzavirus A* (Health Protection Agency 2009). Influenza can occur at any time but is more common during the winter.

Incubation and symptoms

Incubation is generally one to three days with symptoms of fever, muscle aches and pain, malaise, headache, nasal congestion and, in some cases, sore throat and cough.

Prevention

Immunisation protects HCWs, and it must be administered annually as the strains may vary from year to year. Vaccination is guided by WHO guidelines.

Treatment

Influenza is generally self-limiting and, often, no treatment is offered. Antiviral drugs can be prescribed for people at high risk of developing complications. Antiviral drugs reduce the symptoms of influenza when administered within 48 hours of symptom onset (Goering et al 2008, Health Protection Agency 2009). Staff who have influenza must resist the temptation to attend work as this can put other colleagues and patients at risk of catching the infection, which can then develop into other serious conditions, such as pneumonia.

Mycobacterium tuberculosis (TB)

Prolonged close contact with a person infected with TB can result in inhalation of the *M. tuberculosis* bacillus and subsequent infection (Jensen et al 1995). TB infection is initially asymptomatic and remains dormant for years in the lungs of the majority of infected people. People in whom TB results in clinical disease can suffer mild to severe illness which can spread from the lungs as the primary source to various parts of the body, for example bones and kidneys.

HCWs need to maintain heightened vigilance in their standard infection control precautions as multidrug resistant strains of TB are increasing globally. A weakened immune system, for instance as a result of HIV infection, can predispose individuals to TB infection.

Incubation and symptoms

Incubation can be up to a number of years as *M. tuberculosis* bacilli grow very slowly. Most TB symptoms are attributed to an individual's immune responses, therefore they may present variably in infected people although they generally include loss of appetite and weight, and persistent productive or non-productive cough for more than three weeks.

Prevention

Pre-employment screening is important to ensure HCWs are neither predisposed to infection nor a risk to vulnerable patients.

HCWs caring for patients with TB should be immunised with the Bacille Calmette-Guérin (BCG) vaccine prior to commencement of employment if they do not have evidence that they have been immunised, such as the renowned BCG scar, or have a negative Mantoux test.

Care should be taken when looking after patients infected with or suspected to have TB. Correct and appropriate use of respirator masks in accordance with local guidelines should be adhered to. HCWs should be trained in the correct use of respirators.

Treatment

Long-term antimycobacterial drugs are given in varying combinations.

Activity

You have come on duty to commence your shift. You notice that one of your colleagues has a persistent cough, a fever and is sneezing. The colleague informs you that the shift is short of staff due to sickness and therefore the patients have to come first!
- What are the risks to your colleague, the patients, and yourself?
- What actions will you take and why?
- Who will you inform?

Blood-borne viruses

Hepatitis B and C viruses (HBV and HCV) and human immunodeficiency virus (HIV) are the most significant blood-borne viruses. HCWs can be at risk through exposure-prone procedures, such as venepuncture, incisions and suturing. Occupational transmission of blood-borne viruses is commonly through percutaneous (sharps) transmission or after mucocutaneous (splash) exposure of blood or high risk body fluids. Only exposure to body fluid that is potentially infected with a blood-borne virus, for instance blood, breast milk, vaginal secretions, semen, cerebrospinal and peritoneal fluids can transmit these viruses (Department of Health 2007). Urine, faeces and sputum are considered low risk body fluids for the transmission. However, the presence of blood in these fluids may not always be visible, therefore all body fluids should be considered a risk for blood-borne virus transmission.

Visual identification of patients and staff with HBV, HCV and HIV is difficult as many can remain asymptomatic for very long periods. Sharps safety and compliance with appropriate personal protective equipment is critical. Gloves will not prevent sharps injury (Stringer et al 2002). Notably, vinyl gloves have been shown to offer no protection against blood-borne viruses (Infection Control Nurses Association 2002). Broken skin and chronic skin conditions present a high risk of blood-borne virus transmission. These viruses can survive for prolonged periods in the environment at room temperature; HCWs need to be scrupulously aware and careful in dealing with blood contamination of the environment and sharps disposal.

HCWs infected with blood-borne viruses should not be discriminated against and OH departments can offer professional and confidential support, assessments and advice on the management of any blood-borne virus condition, suitability of work or an adjustment of duties if and where necessary.

Inoculation (sharps/needlestick) injuries

Millions of sharps and splash injuries occur globally every year yet most that occur during routine practice are avoidable (Jagger et al 1988, Schaffer 1997, Stringer et al 2002). Scrupulous adherence to standard infection control precautions and sharps safety management, including never re-sheathing needles, is imperative to preventing inoculation injuries (Advisory Committee on Dangerous Pathogens 1990, Gerberding 1990, Puro et al 1995).

Re-sheathing needles is one of the most common causes for sharps injuries and it is essential that this practice is not adopted. The use of safety devices, such as retractable needles or protective sheaths, is ideal.

Sharps containers should always be readily available to ensure that disposal of sharps is prompt and easy at the point of use. Sharps should never be left lying around and never carried away to be discarded elsewhere. Each HCW is responsible for disposing of his or her own sharps; it is unacceptable for the user of a sharp to request or leave sharps to be disposed of by someone else. The entire needle and syringe should be disposed of together as a single unit and not

---

Case study

Healthcare support worker Sally has been working within the infectious disease ward on a busy shift. The doctor has just completed inserting an intravenous catheter into Mrs James, when he is called away to an emergency in the next ward. He asks Sally to help him by clearing the dressing trolley which contains the sharps used for the procedure. Sally wheels the dressing trolley to the clinical room where she notices that the sharps bin is overflowing and sitting near the edge of a shelf.

* What are the risks in this case?
* What actions should Sally take and why?

Key point

* The mantra for all HCWs should be to contact occupational health immediately for any exposure to used sharps or splash injuries

---

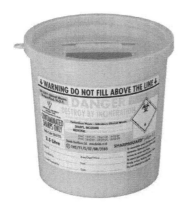

Figure 4.1. Typical sharps bin (published with kind permission from Daniels Healthcare Ltd).

separated since sharps injuries commonly occur at disposal (Jagger et al 1988, Schaffer 1997). The correct sharps container should be used according to local guidelines and, most importantly, HCWs need to know how to assemble, endorse and discard a sharps container correctly. *Figure 4.1* shows a typical sharps bin used within a clinical area.

Davidhizar et al (2000) noted a largely apathetic attitude among nurses in the USA that needlestick injuries do not exist, yet nurses have among the highest incidence of this type of injury (Davidhizar et al 2000, Avert Organisation 2006). There can never be sufficient emphasis on the need for HCWs to understand the dangers posed by reckless handling of sharps and body fluids as well as a disregard of standard infection control precautions.

If exposure to a sharps injury occurs, bleeding should be encouraged immediately, but without sucking. Liberal washing with soap and water should also be carried out straight away, but without scrubbing. Broken skin and mucous membranes should be irrigated immediately with copious amounts of water where the splash has occurred. Contact lenses should be removed if splash occurs in the eyes (Department of Health 2004).

Post-exposure prophylaxis

Occupationally acquired HIV and HBV transmission after sharps and splash injuries can be significantly reduced by post-exposure prophylaxis (Department of Health 2006, World Health Organization 2007). Post-exposure prophylaxis needs to be administered within hours of the exposure even without HIV testing if the risk is high. In the UK, post-exposure prophylaxis is recommended within an hour of exposure (Department of Health 2004) and not longer than 72 hours, as after this time it will no longer be effective. The full course of treatment, where necessary, is for 28 days. However, treatment has low uptake and completion due to adverse side effects such as nausea, diarrhoea and vomiting (Traynor 2005).

Awareness of correct and timely management of occupational exposure to blood-borne viruses is vital. Prompt OH or emergency services advice after a sharps injury ensures that an accurate and timely risk assessment is carried out and, if necessary, post-exposure prophylaxis administered.

In accordance with risk assessments and advice by the occupational health physician, carriers of blood-borne viruses may have to cease performing exposure-prone procedures and have continuous monitoring of their viral loads. Performing exposure-prone procedures may be permitted if the viral load is suppressed to a stipulated level and the HCW remains on antiviral therapy with routine check ups (Puro et al 1995).

Human immunodeficiency virus (HIV)

HIV attacks the immune system and causes acquired immune deficiency syndrome (AIDS). Healthcare workers are far less likely to acquire HIV following a sharps injury than they are of acquiring hepatitis B virus or C virus; however HIV in almost all cases is eventually fatal and often worsened by the stigma and humiliating difficulty of proving that it was contracted through an occupational injury and not high risk behaviour outside of work (Ellis and Symington 1994, Department of Health 2005, Kagan et al 2008).

Incubation and symptoms

HIV is categorised as asymptomatic, symptomatic, or AIDS. Disease progression can range from months to years. Most HIV symptoms are attributed to individuals' immune responses, therefore they may present differently in different infected people. The symptomatic category may include diarrhoea, weight loss and recurrent or frequent opportunistic infections, for example, staphylococcal and herpes virus infections. Persistent generalised enlarged lymph nodes, leukaemia and skin conditions/carcinoma may also present.

Prevention

There is currently no vaccine or cure for HIV although extensive trials are being carried out. It is crucial that HCWs do not expose themselves to the risks of HIV infection, particularly through careless behaviour when dealing with patient's blood and body fluids. All patients should be considered potentially infected with HIV; therefore standard infection control precautions should be used at all times.

Treatment

Prompt post-exposure prophylaxis is vital when occupational exposure occurs, as is lifelong use of antiretroviral drugs if infection occurs.

Hepatitis B viruses

Over 350 million people worldwide are estimated to be chronic carriers of the Hepatitis B viruses (HBV) (World Health Organization 2007). HBV causes progressive liver disease, which can eventually result in liver cirrhosis. Incidences of acute occupational HBV infection are high amongst HCWs. Vaccine is available for HBV and it is administered based on the level of risk.

Incubation and symptoms

Incubation ranges from four to 12 weeks with varying symptoms including:

- upper abdominal pain
- nausea
- jaundice
- malaise
- weight loss
- darker-coloured urine
- lighter-coloured faeces.

Prevention

All HCWs working in high risk clinical areas, such as intensive care and operating theatres, should have the HBV vaccine. Crucially, HCWs should not expose themselves to HBV infection, particularly through careless behaviour when dealing with patient's blood and body fluids.

All patients should be considered as potentially infected with HBV; therefore standard infection control precautions should always be used.

Treatment

Hepatitis B immunoglobulin and immunisation should be administered simultaneously within 48 hours of exposure. Antiviral therapy is prescribed if infection occurs.

Hepatitis C viruses

Hepatitis C viruses (HCV) can be transmitted through occupational exposure to blood via inoculation injuries (Wilson 2006). In the USA, HCV is said to have much higher mortality than AIDS (Tortora et al 2004). HCV often leads to chronic liver disease in which a significant number of people develop liver cirrhosis or cancer. There is currently no vaccine for HCV.

Incubation and symptoms

Incubation ranges from eight to 16 weeks and is generally a subclinical infection, however when symptoms do present they are similar those of HBV.

Prevention

It is crucial that HCWs do not expose themselves to HCV infection, particularly through careless behaviour when dealing with patient's blood and body fluids. All patients should be considered as potentially infected with HCV; therefore standard infection control precautions should always be used.

Treatment

Antiviral treatment is available, although a sustainable response to treatment is relatively rare.

Skin infections and conditions

In this final section we will look at common skin conditions that can affect the HCW within the healthcare setting, namely, infection with the varicella-zoster virus, scabies and also the risk of infection via inflamed and damaged skin caused by dermatitis.

Chickenpox and shingles (varicella–zoster virus)

The primary infection is chickenpox (varicella) which can thereafter lie dormant in the nerve endings and when reactivated due to compromised immunity will present as shingles (zoster). Chickenpox is spread via droplets and contact with saliva or weeping skin lesions, while shingles will be triggered by the individual's own immune system,` although it can be transmitted to those who have not previously had chickenpox infection, via oral secretions. Chickenpox infection can cause complications as well as fetal abnormalities if acquired during early pregnancy.

Incubation and symptoms

Incubation is from two to three weeks. Usually chickenpox presents with a rash that starts on the face or trunk which then spreads rapidly to the limbs. Vesicles, which become pustules, and fever generally occur.

Prevention

Immunity is acquired through previous exposure. If HCWs have not had chickenpox or do not know that they have, they should not nurse patients with chickenpox or shingles. Prompt isolation of infected patients is important and infected staff should stay away, most importantly, when working with immunocompromised patients. Gloves and aprons should be worn when having direct contact with infected patients.

Treatment

Chickenpox and shingles are often self-limiting and no treatment is generally given. Antiviral treatment can be prescribed if there are other high risk factors. These factors can be assessed by the OH department.

Scabies

In scabies an individual's skin is infected by the *Sarcoptes scabiei* mite which is then transmitted by prolonged skin-to-skin contact with a person that does not have the mite. HCWs at risk are often those that have prolonged direct and intimate contact with patients, for instance those caring for the elderly, stroke rehabilitation nursing staff, and physiotherapists. Diagnosis of scabies may be confusing due to scratching of the itching burrows which can result in excoriation and secondary infection of the skin.

Incubation and symptoms

Incubation ranges from four to six weeks with symptoms of itchy rash that develops into papules then vesicles. Lesions appear around the wrists, finger webs, elbows and axillae and also on the abdomen, waist and groin (Health Protection Agency 2009). Shedding of skin scales and scabies mites can occur rarely and only in Norwegian scabies, which is often found in severely immunocompromised people and is generally associated with AIDS.

Prevention

It is necessary to minimise prolonged skin-to-skin contact where possible and ensure the use of appropriate personal protective equipment, e.g. gloves and possibly gowns, where scabies is suspected. The infection control department should be consulted for advice.

Treatment

Treatment consists of a topical insecticide lotion which is applied by staff and their families, who might also have become infected.

Dermatitis

Dermatitis is not an infection, rather an inflammation of the skin due to various causes including sensitivities and allergies to liquid soap and disinfectants. Some HCWs have acquired occupational dermatitis due to latex sensitivity which can be a consequence of glove use. Dermatitis predisposes healthcare workers to infections by opportunistic pathogens, such as some *Staphylococcus* and *Streptococcus* bacteria, blood-borne viruses and fungi. HCWs are at high risk of becoming colonised with various healthcare pathogens such as methicillin-resistant *Staphylococcus aureus* (MRSA).

Immunocompromised HCWs or those on certain types of medication, such as corticosteroids, may be highly susceptible to occupational infections within the clinical environment, depending on their level of exposure and adherence to standard infection control precautions.

Incubation and symptoms

Incubation of skin infections can vary from hours to months depending on the infecting microorganism and tissue affected. Symptoms can include inflamed, sore, itching and irritated skin, dry rashes or un-healing wounds.

Prevention

Use of personal protective equipment should be appropriate and neither under-utilised nor over-used. Good hand care and handwashing technique is essential to ensure that all traces of soap, which can also be an irritant, are thoroughly rinsed off the skin, with the hands dried and moisturised appropriately.

Treatment

The occupational health department should be consulted to assist with a risk assessment and advice on management of such conditions. At times minimising or stopping the affective activity or exposure may be recommended for a period. Emollients, steroids and antimicrobial creams can be used depending on the diagnosis by a specialist or doctor.

Hand hygiene

Good hand hygiene is an integral element of good healthcare provision. Hand washing is the simplest yet one of most important elements in preventing and controlling the spread of infections (Ayliffe et al 1990, Health and Safety Executive 2009), not only for patients but also for the protection of HCWs themselves.

Hands are the biggest cause of healthcare-associated infections, and HCWs' hands are constantly in contact with patients, the patient's environment and other areas of the clinical setting, such as the nurses' station, utility rooms as well as staff rooms. Consequently, resident, transient and any pathogenic organisms on the HCWs' hands are perpetually being transported around all the various areas that HCWs visit during their working period.

The World Health Organization (2009) has highlighted five moments for

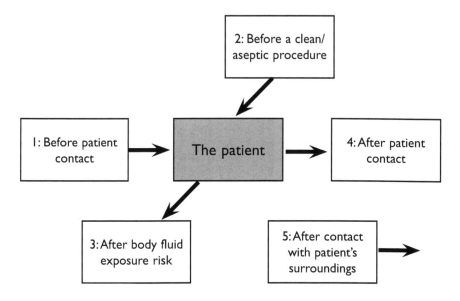

Figure 4.2. The five moments for opportunities to clean hands. (Adapted from World Health Organization 2009)

the opportunity to clean hands. These are critical in reducing the transmission of infections to patients and similarly preventing the HCW taking pathogenic organisms away from patients and their immediate environment to other patients and staff areas (see *Figure 4.2*). Additionally, HCWs need to wash their hands at the beginning and end of every working period, after using or visiting the toilet, and also before handling food or drink in any way, including 'just opening' a drink bottle or chocolate box.

Cursory handwashing is inadequate within a healthcare environment; a specific and precise handwashing technique is paramount for all HCWs. Effective handwashing is a practice that should be mastered promptly (Ayliffe et al 1978, World Health Organization 2009).

HCWs' hands need to be well cared for as chapped skin and sore hands prevent handwashing or the use of alcohol gel because of stinging and discomfort. It is important to prevent skin damage right from the onset through the correct and appropriate use of gloves as well as good moisturising of the hands. Hands should be moisturised when possible with time allowed for the moisture to be absorbed. Water-based and fragrance free hand products are encouraged as the skin will readily absorb the moisture.

To reinforce effective hand washing, the NHS has adopted a 'bare below the

---

A cautionary tale

A first year student nurse conscientiously washed her hands with a solution consisting of 4% chlorhexidene gluconate and decided to add this to a liquid soap in order to ensure the removal of microorganisms from her hands. As both solutions were readily available at every handwash basin, she would continuously put several pumps of both solutions in all her patients' wash water.

The intention here was noble but the action was pointless and potentially problematic.

* The effectiveness of chlorhexidene is reduced by the presence of soap.
* Continuous exposure to sub-optimal levels of chlorhexidine can lead to microbial resistance.

---

elbows' approach, stipulating that HCWs working in any clinical area wear short or rolled up sleeves and no watches, jewellery or gem stone rings. Nail varnish and artificial nails should not be worn and nails should be kept no longer than the finger tips for all clinical HCWs.

The appropriate use of personal protective equipment by HCWs is vital; however, inappropriate use of gloves is endemic due to either lack of understanding, mere carelessness or both. It should be recognised that gloves can have pores in them which will allow microorganisms to pass through and contaminate hands or invade broken skin. Therefore hands should be cleaned before and after wearing gloves (Pratt et al 2007). Wounds and broken skin should be covered adequately with an impermeable dressing to prohibit microorganisms entering the skin and possibly invading deeper tissues or the blood stream. If infection is suspected, help should be sought immediately and the first port of call should be the OH department. Staff should not routinely use nail brushes as these can aggravate the skin. Where nail brushes need to be used, such as in surgery, they should be single use.

Education

Infection prevention and control is virtually impossible if HCWs do not know and understand how infections spread. Education and continuous reinforcement in the form of training updates is essential to embed the importance and methods of infection prevention and control (Sadfar and Abad 2008). Most healthcare organisations have classified infection prevention and control training as mandatory on an annual basis for all clinical staff.

Essentially, all HCWs must undergo induction to the clinical area, which should include hand hygiene, infection control procedures, and how to report adverse incidents, such as sharps injuries with blood contamination. The latter, particularly, is a legal requirement under the Reporting of Injuries, Diseases and Dangerous Occurrences Regulations 1995 (RIDDOR) (Health and Safety Executive 1996).

Healthcare workers in the 21st century are faced with insidious vulnerabilities, from often strenuous shift working patterns, staffing shortages, volatile patients and relatives, to treating and caring for patients with multi-drug resistant infections. Despite this, careful attention must be paid to preventing cross-infection and harm to the patients, colleagues, and self through adhering to consistently high standards of hand hygiene and infection control practices. Furthermore, it is vital that vigilant practice be role modelled for junior staff and students, including staff new to clinical areas.

Summary

In this chapter we have looked at staff health issues, the importance of pre-employment screening and the role of occupational health in helping to safeguard the health of staff. We examined some of the more common infections that staff may be exposed to during the course of their work, and the measures necessary to prevent and treat these. Throughout, we have emphasised best practice around hand hygiene, standard infection control procedures and the importance of staff training and education. In the next chapter we will look at the role of staff in preventing the spread of infection through careful management of the environment.

References

Advisory Committee on Dangerous Pathogens (1990) *Categorisation of pathogens according to hazard and categories of containment* (2nd edn). HMSO, London

Avert Orgnisation (2006) *Healthcare workers and HIV prevention*. Available from http://www.avert.org/needlestick.htm [Accessed 13 March 2010]

Ayliffe GAJ, Babb JR, Quoraishi AH (1978) A test for 'hygienic' hand disinfection. *Journal of Clinical Pathology* **31**: 923–8

Ayliffe GAJ, Collins BJ, Taylor LJ (1990) *Hospital-acquired infection* (2nd edn). Wright, London

Bourdain A (2005) *Typhoid Mary*. Bloomsbury Press, London

Chadwick PR, Beards G, Brown D, Caul EO, Cheesbrough J, Clarke I et al (2000) Management of hospital outbreaks of gastroenteritis due to small round structured viruses. *Journal of Hospital Infections* **45**: 1–10

Davidhizar R, Shearer R, Castro R (2000) Needlestick injury: What every nurse should know. *Journal of Practical Nursing* **Winter**: 12–18

Department of Health (2004) *HIV post-exposure prophylaxis*. Department of Health, London

Department of Health (2005) *HIV infected healthcare workers: Guidance on management and patient notification*. Department of Health, London

Department of Health (2006) *Immunisation against infectious disease*. Department of Health London

Department of Health (2007) *Hepatitis B infected healthcare workers and antiviral therapy*. Department of Health, London

Department of Health (2009) *The Boorman Review of NHS Health and Well-being – A Department of Health response*. Department of Health, London

Ellis CJ, Symington IS (1994) Microbial disease. In Raffle PAB, Adams PH, Baxter PJ, Lee WR (eds) *Hunter's disease of occupations* (8th edn). Edward Arnold, Kent

Health Protection Agency (2009) *Factsheet on scabies*. Available from: http://www.hpa. org.uk/web/HPAwebFile/HPAweb_C/1194947413004 [Accessed 1 May 2010]

Gammon J, Morgan-Samuel H, Gould D (2007) A review of the evidence for suboptimal compliance of healthcare practitioners to standard/universal infection control precautions. *Journal of Clinical Nursing* **17**: 157–67.

Gerberding J (1990) Post HIV exposure management: San Francisco general hospital experience. *AIDS Patient Care* **4**: 22–4

Goering RV, Dockrell HM, Wakelin D, Zuckerman M, Chiodini PL Roitt et al (2008) *Mims' Medical Microbiology* (4th edn). Elsevier, Philadelphia

Health and Safety Executive (1996) *A guide to the Reporting of Injuries, Diseases and Dangerous Occurrences Regulations 1995*. HMSO, London

Health and Safety Executive (2005) *A short guide to the Personal Protective Equipment at work Regulations 1992*. Available from: http://www.hse.gov.uk/pubns/indg174.pdf [Accessed 15 March 2010]

Health and Safety Executive (2009) *Managing skin exposure risks at work*. HSE Books, London

Health Protection Agency (2009) *Swine influenza pandemic (H1N1) 2009 influenza*. Available from: http://www.hpa.org.uk/HPA/Topics/InfectiousDiseases/ InfectionsAZ/1240732817665/ [Accessed 30 March 2010]

Infection Control Nurses Association (2002) *A comprehensive choice of gloves*. Fitwise, Bathgate

Jagger J, Hunt EH, Brand-Elnaggar J, Pearson RD (1988) Rates of needlestick injury caused by various devices in a university hospital. *New England Journal of Medicine* **318**: 284–8

Jensen MM, Wright DN, Robison RA (1995) *Microbiology for the health sciences* (4th edn). Prentice-Hall International, New Jersey

Kagan I, Ovadia KL, Kaneti T (2008) Physicians' and nurses' views on infected healthcare workers. *Nursing Ethics* **15**: 573–85

Madan I, Williams S (2010) *A review of pre-employment health screening of NHS staff.* The Stationary Office, Norwich

NHS Executive (1994) *Occupational Health.* Available from: www.occmed.free-online. co.uk/nohncl/Chap2-7.pdf [Accessed 30 March 2010]

O'Reilly FW, Stevens AB (2002) Sickness absence due to influenza. *Occupational Medicine* **52**: 265–9

Pratt RA, Pellowe CM, Loveday HP et al (2007) Epic 2: National evidence-based guidelines for preventing healthcare associated infections in NHS hospitals in England. *Journal of Hospital Infection* **65S**: S1–64.

Puro V, Petrosillo N, Ippolito G (1995) Italian Study Group on Occupational Risk of HIV and Other Bloodborne Infections. Risk of hepatitis C seroconversion after occupational exposure in healthcare workers. *American Journal of Infection Control* **23**: 273–7

Sadfar N, Abad C (2008) Educational interventions for prevention of healthcare-associated infection: A systematic review. *Critical Care Medicine* **36**: 933–40

Salisbury D, Ramsay M, Noakes K (2006) *Immunisation against infectious disease.* Department of Health, London

Schaffer S (1997) Preventing nursing student exposure incidents: The role of personal protective equipment and safety engineered devices. *Journal of Nursing Education* **36**: 416–20

Stringer B, Infante-Rivard C, Hanley JA (2002) Efffectiveness of the hands-free technique in reducing operating theatre injuries. *Occupational Environmental Medicine* **59**: 703–7

Tortora GJ, Funke BR, Case CL (2004) *Microbiology: An introduction* (8th edn). Benjamin Cummings, San Francisco

Traynor K (2005) HIV occupational exposure guidelines revised. *American Journal of Health-System Pharmacy* **62**: 2332–4

Vagholkar S, Ng J, Chan RC, Bunker J M, Zwar NA (2008) Healthcare workers and immunity to infectious diseases. *Australian and New Zealand Journal of Public Health* **32**: 367–71

Wikipedia (2005) *Mary Malone.* http://en.wikipedia.org/wiki/Mary_Mallon

Wilson J (2006) *Infection control in clinical practice* (3rd edn). Bailliere Tindall, Edinbrugh

World Health Organization (2009) *WHO guidelines on hand hygiene in healthcare: First global patient safety challenge, clean care is safer care.* WHO, Geneva

World Health Organization (2007) *World Health Statistics.* WHO, Geneva

Further reading

Agius R, Seaton A (2006) *Practical occupational medicine* (2nd edn). Hodder Arnold, New York

Alexander MF, Fawcett JN, Runciman PJ (2004) *Nursing practice: Hospital and home. The adult* (2nd edn). Churchill Livingstone, Edinburgh

Aw TC, Gardiner K, Harrington JM (2007) *Pocket consultant occupational health* (5th edn). Blackwell Publishing, Massachusetts

Bierman S (2004) Stamping out risky business. *Managing Infection Control* **4**: 14–20

Centres for Disease Control (1987) Recommendations for the prevention of HIV transmission in healthcare settings. *Morbidity and Mortality Weekly Report* **36**: 2S

Department of Health (1991) *Strategic guide to waste management*. Circular EL (90) M/I. Department of Health, London

Department of Health (2002) *Getting ahead of the curve: A strategy for combating infectious diseases*. Available from: http://www.dh.gov.uk/prod_consum_dh/groups/dh_digitalassets/@dh/@en/documents/digitalasset/dh_4060875.pdf [Accessed 13 March 2010]

Elder AG (2002) Influenza in working populations: An overview. *Occupational Medicine* **52**: 239–40

Litchfield P (1995) *Health risks to the healthcare professional*. Royal College of Physicians of London in association with the Faculty of Occupational Medicine, Salisbury.

Moses CS, Pearson RD, Perry J, Jagger J (2001) Risks to health workers in the developing countries. *New England Journal of Medicine* **345**: 538–40

Pantry S (1995) *Occupational health*. Chapman & Hall, California

Radonovich LJ, Hodgson MJ, Cohen HJ (2008) Do respirators protect health-care workers from airborne infectious diseases? *Respiratory Care* **53**: 1660–4

Ridley J, Channing J (1999) *Safety at work* (5th edn). Butterworth Heinemann, Oxford

Safdar N, Cybéle A (2008) Educational interventions for prevention of healthcare-associated infection: A systematic review. *Critical Care Medicine* **36**: 933–40

Taylor LJ (1978) An evaluation of handwashing techniques. *Nursing Times* **74**: 54–5

Thomas-Copeland J (2009) Do surgical personnel really need to double-glove? *American Operating Room Nurses Journal* **89**: 322–8

Trick WE, Vernon MO, Hayes RA (2003) Impact of ring wearing on hand contamination and comparison of hand hygiene agents in a hospital. *Clinical Infectious Diseases* **36**: 1383–90

CHAPTER 5

Environmental hygiene

Emily Hoban

Purpose

This chapter looks at environmental hygiene in healthcare. It gives an overview of the issues associated with cleaning and decontaminating the environment and discusses ways of addressing the challenges around sustainable solutions for environmental cleanliness. The chapter provides an introduction to the complexities of healthcare cleanliness.

Learning outcomes

By the end of the chapter, you will have learned:

• The key reasons for maintaining a clean environment.
• Methods and strategies for cleaning within the health and social care setting.
• Various types of cleaning equipment in use.
• Different roles and responsibilities in cleaning.

Introduction

If you ask patients what is important when they are receiving treatment within a hospital or any healthcare facility the overwhelming response will be cleanliness. There will be other factors patients consider, such as the medical staff, access and waiting times, but who would want to be treated in an unclean environment? Healthcare workers want to have the best possible environment in which to treat patients and patients want the best possible environment in which to be treated.

It can be a challenge to achieve consistently high standards of cleanliness within a healthcare environment. Cleaning and decontamination are acknowledged as extremely important, but cleanliness needs to be seen as everyone's responsibility, from board to ward, from consultant to cleaner. Everyone has a responsibility to maintain a clean, clutter-free environment.

There are many reasons why high quality cleaning is considered difficult, some of these are outlined in *Box 5.1*.

Box 5.1. Obstacles to maintaining a clean environment

- Processes and systems
- Storage space
- Clutter
- Staff time allocation
- Lack of education/training
- Communication
- Finances
- Everyone thinks it is someone else's job
- Lack of clear management arrangements
- Use of inappropriate techniques

Throughout this chapter, reference is made to key Department of Health and National Patient Safety Agency (NPSA) publications and research carried out linking cleaning to healthcare-associated infections (HCAIs). Although there are some technical aspects to cleaning, fundamentally it is about getting the basics right and everyone having a sense of ownership in maintaining a clean environment.

External regulators of cleanliness

There are external bodies that provide periodic review of the standards of cleanliness within healthcare organisations. These include the Care Quality Commission, that assesses against the Hygiene Code 2008 and specifically criterion 2 (Provide and maintain a clean and appropriate environment in managed premises that facilitates the prevention and control of infection); and Monitor, the regulator for Foundation Trusts, that ensures those Trusts comply with all regulatory requirements, including compliance with healthcare cleanliness and hygiene. The role of the Department of Health is to provide the NHS with regulations, policies and guidance.

Terminology

The most frequently methods of cleaning are shown in *Box 5.2* with details of their different uses in practice in *Box 5.3*.

Box 5.2. Cleaning definitions

- *Cleaning* is the act of making something clean, using either manual methods (cloths, mops and 'physical effort') or mechanical methods (vacuum cleaners, steam cleaners, etc.). In the majority of cases a combination of detergent and warm water is used when cleaning.

- *Cleanliness* is the absence of dirt, dust, debris, stains and clutter following cleaning. Cleanliness reduces the risk of spreading contamination, improves public confidence and promotes a professional image. Cleanliness, however, cannot guarantee an environment free of bacterial contamination. If cleaning is carried out correctly bacterial load will be reduced, but to remove the risk further, specialist cleaning needs to take place, such as disinfection and sterilisation. The choice of method depends on the risk factor of the item being cleaned.

- *Disinfection* reduces bacteria and viruses to safer levels and reduces risk but does not completely destroy and eradicate microorganisms. The disinfection process is usually used when cleaning following an infection on a ward, or when cleaning an item of equipment used by a patient with, or suspected of having, an HCAI. Disinfection is usually chemical, and within a healthcare facility would tend to be a chlorine-based product, alcohol or hydrogen peroxide, although there are many other disinfection products available and appropriate use should be assessed.

- *Sterilisation* is the term used for the complete eradication of bacteria, spores and viruses from a surface or item of equipment. Within healthcare, sterilisation is used to ensure invasive devices, such as surgical instruments are sterile at the point of use. The main method of sterilisation is by moist heat in autoclaves at temperatures ranging from 121°C held for 15 minutes to 134°C held for 3 minutes. Other methods include irradiation, ethylene oxide gas and incineration. Incineration is used to destroy infectious clinical waste.

- *Decontamination* is a combination of processes, including cleaning, disinfection and sterilisation to ensure an item is safe for further use. Effective decontamination is essential to minimise the risk of transmission of infection to patients or staff. The level of decontamination required depends on the level of risk of an individual piece of equipment and this determines its method of cleaning. It is not the case that the decontamination of a piece of equipment always includes sterilisation.

Box 5.3. Use of different cleaning methods in clinical practice

- *Cleaning:* Used to prepare a non-infected bed space after a patient has been discharged
- *Disinfection:* Used to treat medical equipment/appliance such as a commode used between patients
- *Sterilisation:* Used to treat a surgical piece of equipment, such as that used within an operation, e.g. forceps, clamps
- *Incineration:* Used to destroy infectious clinical waste such as removed body tissue, or infected incontinence pads
- *Decontamination:* Used to treat pieces of equipment/medical devices used between patients, e.g. stethoscope, hand washing

---

Key reasons for maintaining high standards of cleaning

There are many reasons to clean, but the two most important are for aesthetic reasons, i.e. everyone wants to be in a clean environment, and hygiene, e.g. to reduce the risk of cross contamination and transmission of potentially harmful microorganisms.

Hospital cleanliness and low rates of infection are selected most often (by 74% of patients) as an important factor when choosing a hospital (Department of Health 2009a). Patients associate a dirty hospital with a high risk of acquiring an infection regardless of scientific evidence. Research looking at the link between a clean environment and infection rates is increasingly showing a close correlation, whereas in the past a link had not been proven (Dancer et al 2009).

Cleaning for aesthetic reasons

How an environment looks and feels is very important for public perception and confidence regardless of where that environment is. If a poor standard of cleanliness and maintenance is experienced within the toilets of a restaurant, for example, confidence in the establishment in providing a safe meal is likely to reduce – what must the kitchens be like? It is highly likely in this case the diner will leave and eat elsewhere.

There has been much media coverage about dirty hospitals over the past 10 years or so, and in the main this is justified. The NHS has come a long way to improve the cleanliness of healthcare establishments, but still public confidence remains low due to continued references to 'dirty hospitals' in the media. However, from a patient's perspective, since 2002, there has been a year-on-year increase in satisfaction with cleanliness in healthcare organisations as evidenced by the Care Quality Commission (CQC) National Inpatient Survey (2009).

An organisation's reputation is extremely important, particularly now that patients are able to choose where they are treated. People want to be treated with dignity. In an unpublished study carried out in the mid-2000s, the overwhelming response to the question about the most important aspect of privacy and dignity was to be treated in a clean environment.

Nobody wants to work in an unclean and cluttered environment. If you work in a clean environment you are more likely to keep it clean and tidy and work in a clean and efficient way. Access to equipment will be easier, there will be confidence that the item is available, that it will be clean when it is needed and that, when it is finished with, it will be cleaned and stored correctly. An orderly environment enables a more efficient way of working. The NHS Institute of Innovation and Improvement has developed a productive ward series (NHS Institute for Innovation and Improvement 2008) that helps to achieve a more efficient working environment. Many organisations who have adopted this systematic approach have benefited by achieving better work flow, better storage and more efficient ordering systems with the outcome of enhanced patient care.

Patient and public confidence in their hospital is extremely important and can be easily undermined by an environment that is unclean or cluttered; and a clean and orderly working environment is equally important for staff. *Box 5.4* outlines other benefits of a clean environment.

Cleaning for infection prevention and control

A number of studies suggest an undefined relationship between cleaning and reducing infection rates. Evidence from case reports and outbreak investigations (Dancer 1999, Garner and Favero 1985) suggest a poor standard of environmental hygiene could be a factor in the transmission of infection. Further evidence shows that the hospital environment can become contaminated with microorganisms associated with HCAIs (Boyce et al 1997, Griffiths et al 2002, Wilcox et al 2003, Barker et al 2004, Denton et al 2004, French et al 2005).

Rampling et al (2001) focused on environmental cleaning to control an outbreak of infection and showed that there is a clear link between the increased number of cleaning hours, with an emphasis on the removal of dust, and the reduction of MRSA.

A further study undertaken by Dancer et al (2009) on a ward at a Glasgow Hospital in 2009 looked at the effect an increase in cleaning frequencies had on the reduction of MRSA. Additional cleaning took place on the 10 most commonly touched surfaces which included patient beds, lockers, tables and call buzzers. The study showed a reduction of 32.5% in microbial contamination on these surfaces. In addition, cases of MRSA fell over the six-month study, but rose once the additional cleaning ceased.

Kiernan et al (2006) showed that *Clostridium difficile* rates increased when targeted cleaning on wards was reduced as staff were reallocated to hospital corridors in order to control dust during a hospital construction phase. When the targeted cleaning resumed on the wards, *Clostridium difficile* levels were once again reduced. Bacterial contaminants can survive in the environment for many months (Kramer et al 2006) and can be found anywhere, on the floors, walls, furniture, equipment and curtains. Both these studies indicate that effective and timely removal of dust and dirt by cleaning is a key defence against the transmission of HCAIs. Dust in the main is made up of human skin cells. With an average person shedding 40–50 thousand skin cells a day, in a hospital ward accommodating many people, both staff and patients, dust control is an important element of the daily cleaning schedule.

Wilcox et al (2003) have shown that shared clinical equipment can become contaminated with bacteria. More than 50% of the commodes tested in a trial determining which was the most effective cleaning product for *Clostridium difficile* infection, were contaminated. This highlights the importance of effective and timely cleaning of commodes between patient use.

Box 5.4. Effective cleaning

Increases
• Confidence of patients and users
• Staff morale
• Reputation of healthcare settings

Decreases
• Risk of infections
• Risk of harm to patients and users

Pratt et al (2007) state that 'good hospital hygiene is an integral and important component of a strategy for preventing healthcare-associated infections in hospitals'.

As more research is performed and evidence gathered, the link between cleaning and the transmission of HCAIs will become clearer.

Standard principles for cleaning

The National Institute for Clinical Excellence (2003) has published standard principles for preventing HCAIs following a review of research and evidence. Those for hospital environmental hygiene are:

- The hospital environment must be visibly clean, free from dust and soilage, and acceptable to patients, their visitors and staff.
- Where a piece of equipment is used for more that one patient (e.g. commode, bath hoist), it must be cleaned following every episode of use.
- Statutory requirements must be met in relation to the safe disposal of clinical waste, laundry arrangements for used and infected linen, food hygiene and pest control.
- All staff involved in hospital hygiene activities must be included in education and training related to the prevention of HCAIs.

Ensuring a clean environment

There are many factors that need to be taken into consideration when setting up a ward or a health and social care environment. *Box 5.5* outlines some of the key issues.

Each of the factors in *Box 5.5* need to be addressed individually and linked together. Effective environmental cleaning and decontamination cannot be one person's responsibility, everyone needs to be involved. Getting the right team together from all departments is key to providing a quality outcome.

Roles and responsibilities

In a report commissioned by Unison, Davies (2009) cites Government policies of the 1980s and 1990s on contracting out domestic services for financial reasons rather than quality and outcome, as a contributory factor to the poor standards of cleanliness within healthcare. The reduction of cleaning cost meant that there was a reduction in the frequency of cleaning as there were fewer domestic cleaners employed, which in turn contributed to a reduction in healthcare cleanliness.

Box 5.5. Key factors in cleaning

- Roles and responsibilities
- Frequency of cleaning
- Scheduling for cleaning
- Cleaning methods
- Risks
- Monitoring and audit
- Training
- Governance
- Assurance

Over the past 10 years the role of the nurse has changed dramatically. Many of the activities carried out today would have been undertaken by doctors in the past. This increase in clinical responsibility has meant a reduction of traditional nursing duties, of which cleaning is just one element.

Both of these factors have led to a reduction in cleanliness in both the environment and equipment due to cleaning frequencies being reduced.

The *NHS Plan* (Department of Health 2000) and subsequent publications, such as the *Matrons' charter* (Department of Health 2004), the *National specifications for cleanliness* (National Patient Safety Agency 2007a), and the *Health Act 2008 Code of practice for the prevention of healthcare associated infections* (Department of Health 2008), have progressively set out the need to have clear lines of responsibility for the management of cleaning and of cleanliness of the environment.

The Health Act 2008 Code of Practice specifically identifies the matron as having overall responsibility for cleanliness on the ward with the nurse in charge of a shift having responsibility of the cleanliness at that time.

The nursing/care and facilities teams within any health and social care setting need to work closely together in order to provide an effective, responsive and efficient cleaning service with the aim of ensuring a clean, safe environment at all times.

Within any healthcare facility, there need to be clear cleaning responsibilities set out, known, understood and documented. There are many formats for a cleaning responsibility matrix, with examples in the *Revised healthcare cleaning manual* (National Patient Safety Agency 2009) and the *National specifications for cleanliness* (National Patient Safety Agency 2007a). Whichever format is used it needs to be clear, easily understood and unambiguous. It needs to identify every item contained in an area and whose responsibility it is to clean it. There are many instances of gaps in cleaning matrices that can result in items of equipment not being cleaned, for example, a visitor chair stacked in a corner of the clinical environment until visiting time. On arrival to the ward, the visitor collects and uses the chair and later returns it to its original position. Who is responsible for cleaning this chair? This is one of many examples where cleaning can be overlooked.

There may be equipment that comes into a healthcare setting that belongs to another department or even another organisation, such as walking frames, wheelchairs and manual handling equipment. Documented procedures need to be in place so that everyone is clear about cleaning these items.

The cleaning responsibility matrix might also include the frequency and method of cleaning.

Within the hierarchical structure of cleaning management, the *National specifications for cleanliness* stipulate that there should be a member of the board who has responsibility for cleanliness of the healthcare facility. This can be the director of nursing, the director of facilities or, in the case of a care home, a member of the senior management team or board. The next level of management is usually an operational manager responsible for environmental cleaning (perhaps a domestic manager) and clinical leaders, such as care managers/team leaders or hospital matrons, for each area who work closely together to ensure a quality cleaning service is delivered. Domestic supervision and supervisors of clinical staff/shifts will be the next tier of staff. Their role is to ensure supervision and monitoring of the cleaning service and output. The nursing and cleaning staff that carry out the majority of the cleaning and decontamination tasks should work closely together to undertake their respective cleaning responsibilities.

The role of the executive lead (e.g. director with responsibility for cleaning)

Box 5.6. Summary of key roles involved in cleaning

- *Executive lead:* Assures the board of the standard of cleanliness
- *Operational lead:* Oversees the implementation of the key actions required for cleanliness
- *Supervisor:* Provides on-the-job support and guidance to staff
- *Front-line staff:* Provide hands on cleaning of equipment and the environment

needs to assure the board on a regular basis that the healthcare organisation is consistently providing a clean environment to maintain a reduction in HCAIs and to increase patient and public confidence.

Frequency of cleaning

Cleaning frequencies must be derived from the application of a risk-based approach of assessing the likelihood of an item causing the transmission of an HCAI to a patient or member of staff. Cleaning frequencies need to be documented and displayed (Department of Health 2008).

Whatever cleaning frequencies are agreed, they will depend not only on risk but also financial constraints. Approximately 90% of most healthcare cleaning budgets are made up of staffing costs, and this may present a challenge for cleaning services during an economic downturn where staffing costs may be reviewed.

Schedules

Once there has is a clear understanding of roles and responsibilities, and cleaning frequencies have been established, the next step is to schedule cleaning activity.

The scheduling of cleaning activity in a health and social care setting cannot be done in isolation; a representative of the ward team and the facilities team must work together in order to get timings right for domestic cleaning. There is no point in a cleaner damp dusting a bay just before the beds are made as dust from the beds will end up in the atmosphere and settle on all those previously dusted surfaces.

Likewise, the scheduling of full toilet and bathroom cleans should not take place at the time patients are getting up as this will mean toilets are out of action when patients are most likely to use them. However, it is important to have some scheduling of toilet cleaning activity at this time just in case an emergency clean is required.

The *National specifications for cleanliness* (National Patient Safety Agency 2007a) and the *Revised healthcare cleaning manual* (National Patient Safety Agency 2009) give examples of cleaning schedules. These can be used to create a user-friendly schedule for the healthcare setting which increases the likelihood of it being more efficient and used by staff.

In addition to documented *domestic* cleaning schedules, there need to be documented *nursing* cleaning schedules. Historically, cleaning of clinical equipment has taken place at the weekend when the clinical areas are quieter but this is becoming increasingly difficult to achieve as healthcare settings become busier. Clear schedules will help to focus effort and act as an aide memoire.

Cleaning risks and methods

Risk factors help to determine the type of cleaning required in a particular area. The *National specifications for cleanliness* identify the risks of a functional area within a healthcare establishment. Commonly there are four levels of risk associated with the area and type of activity, as seen in *Box 5.7*.

Cleaning frequencies and schedules would be based on these risk categories. In addition to cleaning frequencies set against the general risk categories for the area, there may be times when further assessment of risk is needed, particularly in the case of an outbreak of infection. In these cases enhanced or isolation cleaning should be deployed.

Cleaning methods

Disinfection

In the case of cleaning during or following an infection the use of detergent and water is deemed insufficient to reduce bacterial load, so additional disinfection methods are used, such as sodium hypochlorite solution at 1000ppm. Other methods of disinfection such as steam cleaning or hydrogen peroxide vapour could be used.

Box 5.7. Risk categories for clinical areas

- *Low risk*, for example, administration areas
- *Significant risk*, for example, outpatient areas
- *High risk*, for example, general wards/clinical areas
- *Very high risk*, for example, operating theatres, intensive care units

---

Deep cleaning

Deep cleaning is used on a periodic basis, usually annually, depending on the risk in the area. Within the deep clean activity, the ward is usually empty and every item of equipment will undergo thorough cleaning and/or disinfection. The scheduling of this type of clean is paramount; there is a great deal of work required in transferring patients to another area in preparation for a deep clean.

Deep cleaning can also take place on individual items of equipment and could be targeted to specific equipment across the organisation which are deemed a higher risk than other equipment, for example, commodes.

Periodic cleans

Periodic cleans are set regular cleans, such as carpet and curtain cleaning, that are not carried out as part of the normal day-to-day cleaning routine. There is a requirement in the *Health and Social Care Act 2008 Code of practice* (Department of Health 2008) that curtains are changed at regular intervals and that documentary evidence can be shown to this effect. In addition, when a patient is discharged, a clear procedure for ensuring the bed space has been cleaned appropriately is required; this should include all patient hand contact surfaces as identified by Dancer et al (2009) and the mattress. The mattress cover, even though it is waterproof, can be breached due to a needle prick, so unzipping the mattress cover to check the foam for soiling and staining would be considered good practice on patient discharge.

Standard cleaning

Standard cleaning is that which is carried out every day in every part of the organisation. The use of detergent, warm water, cloths and mops are the most common and effective way to clean.

National colour coding for cleaning

The National Patient Safety Agency (2007b) launched a national colour coding system for cleaning. Its aim is to ensure cross-contamination does not occur during the cleaning process. Every healthcare organisation follows the same colour coding scheme, so that when staff move from one place to another there is no confusion, and cross-contamination risk is reduced.

Training

Criterion 9 of the *Health and Social Care Act 2008 Code of practice* (Department of Health 2008) stipulates that there must be a programme of education and training in place for staff in the prevention and control of HCAIs. Training in cleaning methods, products, processes and equipment is extremely important. It is often assumed that someone knows how to clean an item of equipment without training. Cleaning is seen as an unskilled task that anyone can perform, this is not the case, particularly within a complex hospital environment.

Detailed procedures for cleaning equipment and the environment need to be maintained. Staff should be trained in these procedures and their competency assessed at periodic intervals.

In a survey published by the Royal College of Nursing in 2009, 34% of respondents reported that they had received no training in how to clean and decontaminate equipment even though they had a responsibility to undertake this cleaning activity.

In order for cleaning to be effective, training must be carried out commensurate with the individual's level of cleaning responsibility. Doctors should be taught how to clean the equipment they use, for example, stethoscopes, and nursing staff must be trained how to clean equipment they would use, for example, commodes, incubators, blood pressure cuffs, mattresses and so forth. A domestic cleaner must be trained, for example, how to clean floors, bathrooms and beds.

Monitoring and audit

A great emphasis is placed on providing evidence to show cleaning has been undertaken effectively. The *National specifications for cleanliness* (National Patient Safety Agency 2007a) provide a method for measuring cleanliness using the 49-element Audit Sheet. This is the standard measure used within all hospital trusts and is being developed to be applicable to all healthcare organisations from ambulance trusts to GP practices.

This method identifies the frequency of audit and the target cleanliness scores organisations should be achieving, depending on risk category.

Some wards have devised cleaning checklists for patient equipment and many use green tape to show that an item of equipment has been cleaned.

Further audit tools have been developed, such as the High Impact Intervention 8 Care bundle to improve the cleaning and decontamination for patient equipment (Department of Health 2009b). Additional measures, such as adenosine triphosphate (ATP) testing, could also be utilised. This method detects the bacterial load on a surface and is a quick method of assessing the effectiveness of cleaning; however, it does not indicate the bacteria type.

There are different types and levels of monitoring and cleaning audits taking place at any one time. Regular and frequent monitoring and audit is usually carried out by domestic supervisors and ward managers. Periodic auditing is carried out by the facilities manager and matrons. The matron will also carry out an infection control audit, of which environmental cleaning forms a part. On an annual basis the director with responsibility for cleaning will undertake an audit, usually with representation from the patients' group. This annual audit then forms part of the Patient Environment Action Team (PEAT) report which is submitted to the National Patient Safety Agency (NPSA). PEAT is the annual self-assessment of healthcare cleanliness, environment, food, privacy and dignity carried out within healthcare organisations. The NPSA has a responsibility for ensuring patient safety, including the elements featured within the PEAT self-assessments. A proportion of PEAT assessments are externally verified annually.

An annual mattress audit is usually carried by the infection prevention team; however, more frequent checking of mattresses is necessary to ensure the integrity of the waterproof cover. A breach of the waterproof cover will cause seepage of liquid, usually bodily fluids, through to the foam; the foam is then contaminated for future patients using the mattress. Should a mattress be soiled it should be disposed of under the clinical waste policy for the organisation.

Auditing must also include evidence of staff training and could include competency assessment if this is deemed necessary.

Whatever method of audit is used it should provide an accurate reflection of the cleanliness of the environment.

Stop, ask, check...

- Have you received training or an update on how to clean specific pieces of equipment that you use?
- Do you know the polices for cleaning and decontamination within your area?
- Who are the key staff you can approach for further information?
- Are cleaning schedules displayed within your area of work?

Care Quality Commission audit

External audit of an organisation's ability to maintain a safe environment in order to prevent and control HCAIs is carried out by the Care Quality Commission. Following analysis of their published 2009/10 reports on organisations' adherence to the Code of Practice, there are common themes that appear, particularly around cleaning and decontamination. These findings provide vital learning for any organisation and can focus effort in improving cleaning and decontamination services.

Box 5.8 gives some examples of cleaning/decontamination issues raised by CQC in the year 2009/10. To reduce the likelihood these findings occurring again, CQC reports are published and made available to organisations. In addition, healthcare organisations must ensure that all members of staff are aware of their level of cleaning and decontamination responsibility, are fully trained to the required level, and have a pride and take ownership of their environment.

Assurance

Providing assurance for patients, staff boards and regulators that every aspect of cleaning is of the correct standard is essential.

A clear governance structure needs to be in place and there should be clear documentary evidence of the monitoring and auditing that has taken place.

Box 5.8. Key concerns raised by the CQC regarding cleanliness

- Dirty commodes
- Significant dust on surfaces
- Build up of dirt
- Sticky residue left on surfaces
- Soiled mattresses/no system for checking mattresses
- Staff unclear how to clean/decontaminate equipment
- Cluttered store rooms
- Sterile equipment removed from packaging then stored
- No system to identify that equipment has been cleaned

Evidence of corrective actions when failures in cleaning have been observed, together with an assessment of historic patterns and trends in cleaning outcomes in specific risk categories, will show the responsiveness of the trust to deal rapidly with cleaning issues.

A correlation of cleaning results and infection rates could also be a useful method of providing assurance.

Cleaning equipment

Over the last 10 years there has been a rapid advancement in the use of technology in cleaning. Many new manual and mechanical means of delivering a clean and decontaminated environment have been developed. A study carried out by the Department of Health in conjunction with University College Hospital London (2006) looked at the effectiveness of microfibre cloths and steam cleaning technology in the reduction of HCAIs. It concluded that both methods proved very effective at removing microorganisms, dirt and grime and that the use of disinfectant chemicals in all but the most infection-critical areas could be reduced.

Microfibre

Microfibre works by trapping microorganisms into its tightly woven fibres. It is claimed these microorganisms are not transferred to further surfaces due to the structure of the cloth or mop. Research carried out by Hamilton et al (2010) identified that using ultra-microfibre to clean a surface reduced the total viable count (TVC) of microorganisms by 30.2% but when a copper-based biocide was used in conjunction with the microfibre the reduction of TVC was significantly increased to 57.9%. The study also concluded that the use of copper biocide in conjunction with ultra-microfibre gave an immediate antibacterial effect and a longer-term residual antibacterial effect.

Steam cleaning

Steam cleaning uses superheated dry steam at 140°C. It loosens dirt, grease and grime and the high temperatures kill microorganisms. This is known as thermal disinfection. Most steam cleaners will have a vacuum facility that sucks up the dirt, water and contaminant loosened from the cleaned surface and ensures safe removal from the environment.

Hydrogen peroxide vaporisation

Hydrogen peroxide vaporisation is a technique used to disinfect and/or sterilise an area that has been previously cleaned. Its purpose is to remove microorganisms from areas which have been infected by emitting hydrogen peroxide for a pre-determined length of time. It is a hazardous method of disinfection; the area undergoing the treatment needs to be sealed so the vapour does not escape.

Standard cleaning

Standard cleaning methods rely on manual cleaning, including mopping using a variety of mops, either disposable or launderable, and wiping surfaces with cloths. Both these methods require a significant level of training to effectively remove contamination and a good knowledge of cross-contamination.

Other cleaning equipment

Other cleaning equipment includes vacuum cleaners, water extraction machines, scrubbing machines, high speed buffing machines, telescopic tools and carpet shampooers. Further information can be sought from the NPSA's Cleaning Manual (2009).

Whatever cleaning equipment is used, training is required to ensure its effective and safe use.

Estates departments

The role of the estates department must not be overlooked when establishing a system for environmental hygiene. The condition of the building stock, fixtures and fittings has an impact on how the environment can be cleaned. It is very difficult to clean a poorly maintained building, but very easy to clean a new, well-maintained building.

The estate must be maintained appropriately with regular, scheduled planned preventative maintenance activities, with a timely response to repair and maintenance issues.

The fabrics and materials used must be of a high quality, must be able to stand up to the rigors of a busy healthcare environment and must be easy to clean. The design of buildings and refurbishments must take into account infection control requirements including access for effective cleaning.

The use of non-touch equipment is becoming increasingly common within healthcare buildings; this includes no-touch lighting, taps and toilet flushes, all of which can reduce transmission of microorganisms.

The estates department must work in a coordinated way with the infection prevention department, and nursing and domestic staff in order to prevent transmission of infection. One key role of the estates department that can be overlooked is the need to ensure the correct maintenance of the organisation's ventilation systems and ducts.

Ducts, ventilation and humidity

Adequate and appropriate ventilation is important in any building but becomes essential within a healthcare facility. Depending on the type and location of the ventilation system, its purpose is fourfold:

- To control the temperature and humidity of the environment.
- To dilute airborne bacterial contamination.
- To control air movement to reduce the transfer of airborne bacteria.
- To remove unpleasant odours.

There are two main types of ventilation system:

- Natural ventilation.
- Mechanical ventilation.

Natural and mechanical ventilation

Natural ventilation includes windows, doors and associated furniture (grilles, trickle vents, etc.). Mechanical ventilation systems range from stand alone extraction, such as those in toilets and bathrooms, through to specialised air handling units in operating theatres, and systems for isolation facilities.

The type of mechanical ventilation required is determined by the location and use of a particular facility and the risk factors associated with the activity undertaken within the facility.

In a general healthcare environment, such as a ward, a standard ventilation system is usually installed. This will have air input and extract grilles connected by ducts.

In specially designed isolation facilities the ventilation system will be installed to operate with either negative or positive air pressure.

Positive air pressure is used to control outside air entering the area where the patient is being treated. It is used for patients who are immunocompromised, such as transplant patients, and those under going treatment for cancer.

High Efficiency Particulate Air (HEPA) filters are used in positive pressure systems. HEPA filters are densely matted fibres that trap and filter small particles that could re-circulate back into the environment. These particles include mould spores, some bacteria and viruses. A proper HEPA filter is defined by the Institute of Occupational Safety and Health as one that can trap 99.97% of particles 0.3 microns in diameter. A human hair is approximately 50–150 microns in diameter.

Negative pressure systems are installed for the treatment of patients who either have, or are suspected of having, an air-borne infectious disease, such as pulmonary tuberculosis, chickenpox or *Clostridium difficile*. The system works by not allowing air to leave the room when the door is opened, as the air in the room has less pressure than the air outside the room. Many isolation facilities have a secondary door system to further reduce the dispersal of air.

The purpose of ventilation within an operating theatre is to provide clean, conditioned air to ensure the patient is not exposed to airborne bacterial contamination which could cause infection within the wound site. Ventilation also assists in the dilution and removal of waste anaesthetic gases, particularly within maternity theatres. Both positive pressure ventilation and air exchange are used in these environments. Department of Health (2003) guidelines identify the number of air changes per hour, optimal air temperature and optimal humidity, depending on the type of procedure being carried out.

Cleaning and maintenance of ventilation systems

In order for air handling and ventilation systems to be effective in the removal of bacteria and the conditioning of air, they must be correctly installed and maintained.

If the ventilation system is not adequately maintained, it has been shown that the system itself can be a vehicle for the transmission and spread of airborne bacteria (Chow et al 2003, Chow and Yang 2004). Not only can the system be a vehicle in contamination, it can also be a cause for contamination. Lack of appropriate cleaning and maintenance of the internal works, ducts and grilles can lead to the growth of organisms such as MRSA, *Clostridium difficile* and *Legionella* which can subsequently be transferred and contaminate the environment. This can occur if:

- The temperature and humidity of the system is incorrectly maintained.
- There is a reduction in the efficiency of the filters.
- The system is not regularly cleaned resulting in a build up of dust and debris.

Routine maintenance must be performed by an appropriately trained engineer. However, certain maintenance activities can be carried out by ward/departmental staff and cleaning staff. These activities, in the main, include the removal of dust, dirt and debris from input and extraction grilles. These are very important components of the maintenance schedule and as such should be documented within it with clear responsibilities understood and appropriate training given.

Any maintenance activities on the ventilation system which will affect the running of the department must be scheduled in conjunction with the operational workload of that department. For example, an emergency operating theatre cannot be shut down for maintenance before alternative arrangements have been planned.

Air sampling and microbiological testing are not usually regular maintenance activities. However, it is important following commissioning of a new installation, if a system has been shut down for maintenance, or if there is a suspected epidemiological link to an outbreak of an airborne infection.

A holistic approach to cleaning

Although there is a low level of evidence to support the link between cleaning and reducing infection rates, this is principally due to lack of research in this area

---

Box 5.9. Points to remember about ventilation

- Ventilation controls temperature and humidity and dilutes and/or removes airborne bacterial contamination
- The two types of ventilation systems are natural and mechanical
- Positive pressure systems ensure air does not enter a room, often used for immunocompromised patients
- Negative pressure systems ensure air does not leave a room, may be used for patients with infectious disease
- The cleaning of all types of ventilation system is important to ensure its efficiency and reduce the risk of the growth of organisms such as legionella

rather than clear evidence to refute the link. Cleaning and decontamination are seen as important in the fight against HCAIs. Additionally, a clean environment is a key factor in improving patients' confidence in healthcare and the services provided.

Cleaning is not just something cleaning staff do, cleaning is everyone's responsibility from board to ward; doctors should clean their stethoscopes between patients, engineers should clean ventilation ducts, administrators should clean their desks, nurses should clean commodes between patients, and cleaners should clean the environment daily.

A whole-system, holistic approach to cleaning is required when managing environmental hygiene and many facets need to be joined together. There are many different levels of responsibility within the organisation and a clear knowledge of roles and responsibilities is required to ensure all environmental hygiene, cleaning, and decontamination activities are managed jointly, appropriately and effectively to provide a clean, safe environment for patients, visitors and staff.

Summary

This chapter has looked at the general principles around cleaning a health and social care environment. It has discussed the roles and responsibilities of the staff involved, and highlighted some of the technologies in place. It also looked at best practice required to reduce the risk of infection to patients and service users and to improve their confidence and experience. In the next chapter we will look specifically at the decontamination of medical equipment used within healthcare settings.

Case study

Mr Jones has been transferred to another hospital. Whilst in your department he was cared for in an open ward until he developed diarrhoea and symptoms of tuberculosis.
- How should the area be cleaned in order to prevent cross-infection to other patients/clients?
- What actions should be taken with his mattress, curtains and medical equipment?

References

Barker J, Vipond IB, Bloomfield SF (2004) Effects of cleaning and disinfection in reducing the spread of *Norovirus* contamination via environmental surfaces. *Journal of Hospital Infection* **58**: 42–9

Boyce JM, Potter-Bynoe G, Chenevert C, King T (1997) Environmental contamination due to methicillin-resistant *Staphylococcus aureus*: possible infection control implications. *Infection Control and Hospital Epidemiology* **18**: 622–7

Care Quality Commission (2009) *National Inpatient Survey*. Available from: http://www.cqc.org.uk/usingcareservices/healthcare/patientsurveys/hospitalcare/inpatientservices.cfm [accessed 31 March 2010]

Chow TT, Lin Z, Yang XY (2003) Study of air infection risk in operating theatre. *Proceedings of Healthy Building 2003, the 7th International Conference, Singapore* **3**: 643–8

Chow TT, Yang XY (2004) Ventilation performance in operating theatre against airborne infection: Review of research activities and practical guidance. *Journal of Hospital Infection* **56S**: 85–92

Dancer SJ (1999) Mopping up hospital infection. *Journal of Hospital Infection* **43**: 85–100

Dancer SJ, White LF, Lamb J, Girvan, EK, Robertson C (2009) Measuring the effect of enhanced cleaning in a UK hospital: A prospective cross-over study. *BMC Medicine* **7**: 28

Davies S (2009) *Making the connections, contract cleaning and infection control.* Unison, Cardiff University

Department of Health (2000) T*he NHS Plan: A plan for investment and plan for reform.* Available from: http://www.dh.gov.uk/en/Publicationsandstatistics/Publications/PublicationsPolicyAndGuidance/DH_4002960 [accessed 2 April 2010]

Department of Health (2003) *HFN 30: Infection control in the built environment.* Available from: https://estatesknowledge.dh.gov.uk/index.php?option=com_documents&Itemid=1&sdocid=150 [accessed 31 March 2010]

Department of Health (2004) *A matron's charter, an action plan for cleaner hospitals.* Available from: http://www.dh.gov.uk/en/Publicationsandstatistics/Publications/PublicationsPolicyAndGuidance/DH_4091506 [accessed 2 April 2010]

Department of Health (2006) *An integrate approach to hospital cleaning: Microfibre cloth and steam technology.* Available from: www.ahcp.co.uk/openarea/microfibrereport3dh.pdf [accessed 31 March 2010]

Department of Health (2007) *Chief Nursing Officers letter PL/CNO (2007)6, Improving Cleanliness and Infection Control*. Available from: http://www. dh.gov.uk/en/Publicationsandstatistics/Lettersandcirculars/Professionalletters/ Chiefnursingofficerletters/DH_080053 [accessed 31 March 2010]

Department of Health (2008) *The Health and Social Care Act 2008 Code of Practice for the prevention and control of healthcare associated infections and related guidance*. Available from: http://www.dh.gov.uk/en/Publicationsandstatistics/Publications/ PublicationsPolicyAndGuidance/DH_4139336 [accessed 2 April 2010]

Department of Health (2009a) *Report of the National Patient Choice Survey, England - December 2008*. Department of Health, London

Department of Health (2009b) *High Impact Intervention No 8 Care bundle to improve the cleaning and decontamination for patient equipment*. Available from: http://www. clean-safe-care.nhs.uk/Documents/High_Impact_Intervention_No_8.pdf [accessed 2 April 2010]

Denton M, Wilcox MH, Parnell P, Green D, Keer V, Hawkey PM, Evans I, Murphy P (2004) Role of environmental cleaning in controlling an outbreak of Acinetobacter baumannii on a neurosurgical unit. *Journal of Hospital Infection* **56**: 106–10

French GL, Otter JA, Shannon KP, Adams NMT, Watling D, Parks MJ (2004) Tackling contamination of the hospital environment by methicillin-resistant *Staphylococcus aureus* (MRSA): A comparison between conventional terminal cleaning and hydrogen peroxide vapour decontamination. *Journal of Hospital Infection* **57**: 31–7

Garner JS, Favero MS (1985) CDC Guideline for handwashing and hospital environmental control. *Infection Control* **7**: 231–5

Griffiths R, Fernandez R, Halcomb E (2002) Reservoirs of MRSA in the acute hospital setting: A systematic review. *Contemporary Nurse* **13**: 38–49

Hamilton D, Foster A, Ballantyne, L, Kingsmore P, Bedwell D, Hall TJ, Hickok SS, Jeanes A, Coen PG, Gant VA (2010) Performance of ultramicrofibre cleaning technology with or without addition of a novel copper-based biocide. *Journal of Hospital Infection* **74**(1): 62–71

Kiernan M, Bowley JA, Jukka C (2006) The effect of construction work on *Clostridium difficile* following short term reallocation of hospital cleaning teams. *Journal of Hospital Infection* **64**(1): S47

Kramer A, Schwebke I, Kampf G (2006) How long to nosocomial pathogens persist on inanimate surfaces? A systematic review. *BMC Infectious Disease* **6**: 130

National Institute for Clinical Excellence (2003) *Infection Control: Prevention of healthcare associated infection in primary and community care*. NICE, London

National Patient Safety Agency (2007a) *National specification for cleanliness in the NHS*. Available from: http://www.nrls.npsa.nhs.uk/resources/?entryid45=59818 [accessed 31 March 2010]

National Patient Safety Agency (2007b) *Colour coding hospital cleaning materials and equipment*. Available from: http://www.nrls.npsa.nhs.uk/resources/?EntryId45=59810 [accessed 31 March 2010]

National Patient Safety Agency (2009) *Revised healthcare cleaning manual*. Available from: http://www.nrls.npsa.nhs.uk/resources/?EntryId45=61830 [accessed 31 March 2010]

NHS Institute for Innovation and Improvement (2008) The productive ward: Releasing time to care. NHS Institute for Innovation and Improvement, London

Pratt RJ, Pellowe CM, Wilson JA, Loveday HP, Harper PJ, Jones SRLJ, McDougall C, Wilcox MH (2007) Epic 2: National evidence-based guidelines for preventing healthcare associated infections in NHS hospitals in England. *Journal of Hospital Infection* **65**: S1–S64

Rampling A, Wiseman S, Davis L, Hyett AP, Walbridge AN, Payne GC, Cornaby AJ (2001) Evidence that hospital hygiene is important in the control of methicillin-resistant *Staphylococcus aureus*. *Journal of Hospital Infection* **49**: 109–16

Royal College of Nursing (2009) *Healthcare staff must have the time and resource to clean*. Available from: http://www.rcn.org.uk/newsevents/news/article/uk/rcn_health_care_staff_must_have_the_time_and_resources_to_clean [accessed 31 March 2010]

Wilcox MH, Fawley WN, Wigglesworth N, Parnell P, Verity P, Freeman J (2003) Comparison of the effect of detergent versus hypochlorite on environmental contamination and incidence of *Clostridium difficile* infection. *Journal of Hospital Infection* **54**: 109–14

Further reading

Association of Healthcare Cleaning Professionals website: http://www.ahcp.co.uk/

Department of Health and the Health Protection Agency (2009) *Clostridium difficile: How to deal with the problem*. Available from: http://www.dh.gov.uk/en/Publicationsandstatistics/Publications/PublicationsPolicyAndGuidance/DH_093220 [accessed 2 April 2010]

Department of Health (2007) *HTM 01 01 Decontamination of reusable medical devices*. Department of Health, London

Department of Health (2006) *HTM 07 01 Safe management of healthcare waste*. Department of Health, London

Department of Health (2006) *Standards for better health*. Available from: http://www. dh.gov.uk/en/Publicationsandstatistics/Publications/PublicationsPolicyAndGuidance/ DH_4086665 [accessed 2 April 2010]

Department of Health (2004) T*owards cleaner hospitals and lower rates of infection*. Available from: http://www.dh.gov.uk/en/Publicationsandstatistics/Publications/ PublicationsPolicyAndGuidance/DH_4085649 [accessed 2 April 2010]

Royal College of Nursing and the Infection Prevention Society (2009) I*nfection prevention and control minimum standards*. Available from: http://www.rcn.org.uk/downloads/publications/public_pub/002725.pdf [accessed 2 April 2010]

CHAPTER 6

Decontamination of reusable surgical instruments

Louise Hodgson

Purpose

This chapter outlines the complex process that involves several decontamination stages which are required to render reusable surgical instruments safe for further use. It explores specialist decontamination methods and equipment and the facilities required.

Learning outcome

By the end of the chapter, you will have learned:

- The principles of safe practices for decontaminating reusable instruments.
- An overview of decontamination methods.
- The decontamination life cycle.
- Microbiological activity of decontamination.

Introduction

Under the Health and Social Care Act,

> *Healthcare organisations are required to provide a safe decontamination service that generates a clean and sterile product. At the core of the service must be a culture committed to successful clinical outcomes and the well-being of patients and staff.*

(Department of Health 2006)

The *Guide to the decontamination of reusable surgical instruments* (NHS Estates 2003a) reports the need to minimise the risk of transmission of infectious organisms. As a result, effective decontamination of reusable surgical instruments is essential.

Challenges around decontamination of instruments

Over the last 10 years there has been a vast amount of work undertaken to improve decontamination standards. A sample survey of NHS decontamination services in 1999 (NHS Estates 2000) found instances where decontamination processes fell short of current standards. In some cases, practice was poor, leading to cross-infection between patients or between patients and staff. The survey identified substantial improvements that could be achieved by effective management of decontamination systems and staff development and training, but also found that much of the buildings and equipment supporting decontamination operations (sterile services departments) needed refurbishment or replacement.

A decontamination programme, the *Strategy for modernising the provision for decontamination services,* was undertaken (NHS Estates 2003b). The perceived major risk of infection transmission highlighted was by surgical instruments (NHS Estates 2000) and these decontamination improvement policies focused on secondary or acute services. The duty of care to all patients and staff crosses boundaries into all sectors of healthcare. Healthcare-associated infection (HCAI) exists in primary care as well as secondary and tertiary care sectors (Department of Health 2007). Therefore, other healthcare service providers such as general medical and dental services in primary care also have to ensure that they comply with Department of Health policy. In practice this means there is a need to have in place modern services and, where relevant, facilities that ensure decontamination is achieved in compliance with current Department of Health policy. This will ensure that the quality and safety of reprocessed or single use products is equal across all sectors (Department of Health 2007).

Lessons from Creutzfeldt-Jakob disease (CJD)

Creutzfeldt-Jakob disease (CJD) belongs to a group of diseases called transmissible spongiform encephalopathies which can occur in people or animals. The diseases are characterised by degeneration of the nervous system and are invariably fatal. The Spongiform Encephalopathy Advisory Committee (SEAC) advises that a key factor in reducing the risk of person-to-person spread during surgery is to ensure that high standards of decontamination of surgical instruments are maintained (NHS Estates 2003a).

The National Institute for Health and Clinical Excellence (NICE 2006) produced guidance entitled *Patient safety and reduction of risk of transmission of Creutzfeldt-Jakob disease (CJD) via interventional procedures.* The

---

Box 6.1. NICE recommendation for the reduction of risks of transmission of CJD via interventional procedures

- Steps should be taken urgently to ensure that instruments in contact with high-risk tissues do not move from one instrument set to another
- Supplementary instruments that come into contact with high-risk tissues remain with the set to which they have been introduced
- Rigid rather than flexible neuroendoscopes should be used wherever possible
- All accessories used through neuroendoscopes for interventions such as biopsies should be single use
- A special separate pool of reusable surgical instruments and new neuroendoscopes for high-risk procedures should be used for children born after 1st January 1997
- Apart from neuroendoscope accessories, the guidance does not advocate a wholesale move to single use instruments and specifically advises that single use instruments should only be used if they are of equivalent quality to reusable instruments

---

recommendations relate to those instruments that have or may have come into contact with high-risk tissues, defined primarily as brain and posterior eye. The main recommendations are outlined in *Box 6.1*.

In addition to this, some dental instruments have also been identified as posing a risk of variant CJD (vCJD) as they are difficult to clean. These instruments are endontic files and reamers and it is recommended that they are single use (Department of Health 2009). To support this, further studies have shown a wide variation in the quality and methods used to clean endontic files and reamers in general dental practice with a large proportion showing visual evidence of contamination after cleaning (Department of Health 2007).

Surgical instruments are used in both the primary and hospital settings, for example, within an operating theatre, a dental surgery, a GP practice or a podiatry clinic. Surgical instruments are either:

- re-usable: the decontamination process is undertaken after its use, or
- single use: the instrument is used once and discarded.

The decontamination of instruments is undertaken either in a specialised unit, a sterilisation services department, or within the healthcare setting, for example, in a general dental practice which is compliant with national standards/regulations.

Decontamination methods

The term decontamination describes the combination of the following processes:

* Cleaning
* Disinfection
* Sterilisation (sometimes described as reprocessing).

The decontamination method required depends on the infection risk of the instrument; *Table 6.1* outlines this further (Medicines Devices Agency 2002).

In order to reprocess a surgical instrument the decontamination method required is sterilisation, as stated in *Table 6.1*, as this item would be in close contact with a break in the skin or mucous membranes and can be introduced into body areas. However, before an instrument is sterilised it must be cleaned and disinfected first. Therefore surgical instruments require all the processes: cleaning, disinfection and sterilisation.

The Department of Health (2009) reports that the decontamination of instruments (reprocessing) is a complex process that involves several stages, including cleaning, disinfection, inspection and a sterilisation step. It goes further to suggest that, prior to sterilisation, cleaned instruments should be free of visible contamination, irrespective of the technology used for cleaning. Instruments

Table 6.1. Choice of decontamination method according to risk

Risk	Application of item	Recommendation
High	• In close contact with a break in the skin or mucous membrane • Introduced into sterile body areas	• Sterilisation required
Intermediate	• In contact with mucous membranes • Contaminated with particularly virulent or readily transmissible organisms • Prior to use on immunocompromised patients	• Sterilisation or disinfection required • Cleaning may be acceptable in some agreed situations
Low	• In contact with healthy skin • Not in contact with patient	• Cleaning

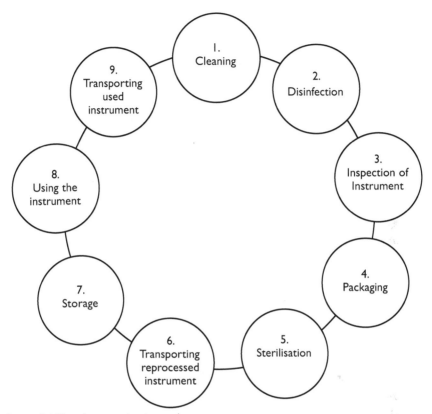

Figure 6.1. The decontamination cycle.

should be reprocessed using a validated decontamination method. The cycle includes: cleaning/washing and sterilisation using a validated steam steriliser. At the end of the reprocessing cycle, the instrument should be in a sterilised state (Department of Health 2009).

This complex process has been described as the decontamination life cycle (NHS Estates 2003b). The processes of the cycle are outlined in *Figure 6.1* and will be discussed in more detail below.

In order to undertake effective decontamination, as reported in the NHS Estates document (NHS Estates 2003a), all these stages of the cycle must be met to an acceptable standard, and any failure to address issues that may impact on the cycle at any of the stages will result in inadequate decontamination.

NHS Estates also advises that at all stages of reprocessing the following issues need to be taken into account:

101

- The location and activities where decontamination takes place.
- Facilities and equipment at each location.
- Assurance that equipment used is validated, maintained and tested in accordance with manufacturers' guidelines and legislation.
- The existence of effective management arrangements.
- The existence of policies and procedures for all aspects of decontamination work.

The next section of the chapter outlines processes of the life cycle, starting with cleaning.

Cleaning

The beginning of the decontamination process for an instrument is cleaning.

Cleaning is a process which physically removes infectious agents and the organic matter on which they thrive but does not necessarily destroy infectious agents. The reduction of microbial contamination depends upon many factors, including the effectiveness of the cleaning process and the initial bioburden. Cleaning is an essential prerequisite to ensure effective disinfection or sterilisation.

(Medicines Devices Agency 2002)

The cleaning of instruments can be undertaken by hand or by using an automated process, the latter being preferable (NHS Estates 2003a).

Manual cleaning

There may be some instances where manual cleaning is acceptable; for example, if the manufacturer's instructions specify that the device is not compatible with automated processes. Manual cleaning is not the preferred method due to the difficulty in ensuring the risk of inoculation, splashing of the healthcare worker and the inability of validating the effectivity of the process.

For manual cleaning of instruments, a double decontamination sink should be used, one with a specialist detergent and warm water and the other with clean water to rinse the instruments. Brushes and clothes are used to clean the instruments.

Washer-disinfectors

Washer-disinfectors undertake the automated process of cleaning and then disinfection. Each stage of the decontamination process enables the reduction of bio-burden on the device being reprocessed. The recognised stages of the washing process may include a cool pre-wash (below 35°C to prevent protein coagulation), main wash, rinse, thermal disinfection and, where appropriate, post-disinfection rinse (NHS Estates 2003a).

Ultrasonic cleaners

Ultrasonic cleaners use an agitation process to remove soil. They may either clean only (ultrasonic bath) or clean and disinfect (washer-disinfectors).

Ultrasonic baths are still used in some primary care settings. Potable water (drinking quality) and a measured amount of detergent, as per manufacturer's instructions, is used as the cleaning/disinfection agent. This method of cleaning should be seen as a first-stage cleaning process, which would normally be followed by cleaning in a washer-disinfector or, where this is unavailable, a thorough rinse before sterilisation (Perry 2007). It is vital that practices are in line with the European guidelines for decontamination and other national regulations, such as those produced by NHS Estates (2003b).

Personal protective clothing, such as gloves, aprons and eye protection, should be worn for manual cleaning and the handling of chemicals. Robust rubber gloves should also be worn to protect the hands when handling sharp instruments/ chemicals.

Disinfection

The next stage of the process is disinfection, which is used to reduce the number of viable infectious agents but which may not necessarily inactivate some microbial agents, such as certain viruses and bacterial spores.

Disinfection does not achieve the same reduction in microbial contamination levels as sterilisation.

(Medicines Devices Agency 2002)

This process reduces the number of organisms further than cleaning but is not effective against some viruses and spores.

The use of moist heat or liquid chemicals are the most common methods of disinfection. Of the two, moist heat is the preferred method as not only is it easily controlled but it tends not to leave any chemical residue on the instruments (NHS Estates 2003a). As previously discussed, most washer-disinfectors incorporate a disinfection stage.

A chemical disinfectant can be defined as

...a compound or mixture which, under defined conditions, is capable of destroying microorganisms by chemical or physico-chemical means.

(Medicines Devices Agency 2002)

The chemical disinfectant can either take the form of a liquid (which is its usual form), or a gas. Within clinical areas, disinfectants are sometimes supplied ready for use. However, it is not usual to find some that need to be diluted in order to attain the correct strength for use. As disinfectants vary in their properties, it is vital that the instructions for use are adhered to. The choice of disinfectant is made in line with national and local policies, as is its storage and disposal.

Inspection

All instruments that have been through any cleaning procedure, including processing by a washer-disinfector, should be inspected to ensure they are clean, functional and in good state of repair (Department of Health 2007). A magnifying lamp is often used to inspect the instruments.

Packaging

It is not always necessary for instruments to be wrapped before being sterilised, i.e. instruments reprocessed in non-vacuum bench-top or bowl and instrument sterilisers. Packaging is not recommended by NHS Estates (2003a) as it may hamper the penetration of steam to all surfaces of the instrument and as a result inhibit sterilisation from occurring.

In porous load/vacuum sterilisers, NHS Estates (2003a) outlines the following reasons for packaging instruments:

- To contain the product through the different stages of the decontamination process.

- To allow sterilisation to take place.
- To protect the product during sterilisation and transportation from deterioration and damage.
- To maintain sterility to the point of use.
- To prevent re-contamination of the product following decontamination.

Sterilisation

The final step in the decontamination process is sterilisation. As previously mentioned, items must first be thoroughly cleaned and disinfected prior to sterilisation for the process to be effective. Validated sterilisation involves complete destruction of all microorganisms, even including spores that are notoriously difficult to destroy. The preferred method within the clinical setting is the use of high temperature saturated steam. This is delivered under pressure, but consideration must be given to its compatibility with the product requiring sterilisation.

A number of different types of steriliser are used within the healthcare setting:

- *Porous-load sterilisers*: These are steam autoclaves with an active air removal stage designed to process wrapped goods or lumened devices.
- *Bowl and instrument sterilisers*: These machines often have large capacity and may be found in operating theatres. They have cycle parameters similar to those of porous load sterilisers but without an active air-removal stage or drying cycle, therefore prohibiting packaged loads from being sterilised. Their use is limited to sterilising items that are solid and not hollow or cannulated.
- *Bench-top steam sterilisers*: There are several types available. The two most common are:

Stop, check, ask...

- All disinfection process must be in line with the EU guidelines and national policy
- What is the policy for decontamination within your local area?
- What action will you take if you have a concern around decontamination?
- Who will you contact?

- Non-vacuum (type N): Commonly used for surgical instruments that are unwrapped, not hollow and do not have lumens.
- Vacuum (type B): Can be used for wrapped and hollow/lumen instruments.

Microbiological activity of decontamination

Table 6.2 outlines the microbiological activity of the decontamination methods. Please note cleaning is not included in the table as it physically removes infectious agents without necessarily destroying them.

Table 6.2. Microbicidal activity of decontamination methods. From MAC manual: Part I (Medical Devices Agency 2002)				
	Spores	*Mycobacteria*	*Bacteria*	*Viruses*
Disinfection				
Thermal washer-disinfector	x	√√√	√√√	√√
Low temperature steam	x	√√√	√√√	√√
Chemical disinfectant				
Alcohol	x	√√	√√√	√√
Glutaraldehyde	√	√√√	√√√	√√√
Ortho-phthalaldehyde	√	√√√	√√√	√√√
Other aldehydes	√	√√√	√√√	√√√
Chlorine dioxide	√√√	√√√	√√√	√√√
Peracetic acid	√√√	√√√	√√√	√√√
Other peroxygen compounds	x	√	√√√	√√
Quaternary ammonium compounds	x	√√	√√	√√
Superoxidised saline	√√√	√√√	√√√	√√√
Sterilisation				
Steam	√√√	√√√	√√√	√√√
Dry heat	√	√	√	√
Gas plasma	√√√	√√√	√√√	√√√
Key: x none, √ poor, √√ moderate, √√ moderate, √√√ good				

Box 6.2. Recommended requirements for transport of containers

- Leak-proof: To reduce likelihood of cross infection
- Easy to clean: To help reduce infection risk
- Capable of being closed securely: To prevent loss or damage
- Lockable (where appropriate): To prevent tampering
- Clearly labelled: To identify the user and the contents
- Robust: To prevent instruments being damaged in transit
- Rigid: To contain instruments and prevent them becoming a sharps hazard to anyone handling the goods and to protect them against accidental damage

(NHS Estates 2003a)

Transport of used instruments

All used surgical instruments present a risk of infection and to minimise this risk, the instruments must be placed in closed, secure containers and transported to the decontamination area as soon as possible following use. Transport containers must protect both the product during transit and the handler from inadvertent contamination. *Box 6.2* lists the requirements of such containers.

Storage

When storing instruments it is vital that recontamination does not occur. The storage conditions must allow the maintenance of the packs/instruments in the condition in which they are required for use. Sterile products are usually stored at the point of use, for example treatment rooms, wards, clinics, care homes, departments and operating theatres (NHS Estates 2003a). The storage area must be dedicated for that purpose and not used for other activities, such as patient treatment.

Within these areas, the storage facilities should be appropriately designed to prevent damage to packs and to allow for the strict rotation of stock. Shelving should be easy to clean and should allow the free movement of air around the stored product.

Products must be stored above floor level, away from direct sunlight and water, in a secure, dry and cool environment (NHS Estates 2003a).

Decontamination facilities

The decontamination of instruments is likely to take place in the following places.

Sterile service department (SSD)

Within the SSD, instruments from a variety of clinical departments in the acute hospital setting or primary care are reprocessed. This process involves the surgical instrument being collected from the client, cleaned/sterilised and then returned.

Local reprocessing units

These occur in dental practices in the primary care setting; only instruments from within that practice are decontaminated before re-use. It is important to note that the premises and facilities must be compliant with the national guidelines.

Decontamination in a general dental practice

Compliance with the Department of Health decontamination programme in general dental practices was considered by some practices to be a challenge due to the complexity of the instruments used and cost factors. Therefore, specialised guidance was published by the Department of Health (2009). This is likely to facilitate best practice within this clinical area.

Regardless of where the decontamination is carried out, the risk of recontamination of instruments must be minimised.

Tracking and traceability of surgical instruments

It is important to be able to trace products through the decontamination processes to which they have been subjected and also to be able to trace the patient on whom they have been used. The ability to track and trace surgical instruments and equipment through the decontamination life-cycle enables corrective action to be taken when necessary. For example, in the unlikely event of a sterilisation cycle failure, products can then be recalled (NHS Estates 2003a).

Records should be maintained for all the sets of surgical instruments cleaned, identifying:

- The cleaning and sterilisation method used.
- The name of the person undertaking the decontamination.
- Details of the actual item being processed.

This information is required so that instrument sets can be traced, if required, in the event of a failure in the decontamination cycle or for infection control reasons. Records relating to decontamination processes should be maintained by the organisation for a minimum of 11 years or in accordance with local policies (NHS Estates 2003a).

Case study

Staff Nurse Jones has been asked to undertake an aseptic technique procedure on Mrs Peters. On setting up the clinical trolley, she finds the dressing pack has a hole in it. She also notes that this is the last pack of its kind on the ward, and the stores delivery is not due until later the next day.
- Based on your learning from this chapter, what actions should Staff Nurse Jones take?
- What are the hazards of using the damaged dressing pack?

Summary

This chapter has looked at some challenges around the decontamination of surgical instruments and the vital steps required to safeguard best practice. It has provided an overview of some key sterilisation methods and looked in detail at the decontamination cycle. In the next chapter we will look specifically at protective measures that can be used to further safeguard patients, staff and visitors to health and social care settings.

References

Department of Health (2006) *The Health Act 2006: Code of practice for the prevention and control of healthcare associated infections.* Available from: http://www. dh.gov.uk/en/Publicationsandstatistics/Publications/PublicationsPolicyAndGuidance/ DH_081927 [accessed 13th March 2010]

Department of Health (2007) *Letter to the Chief Executive of the British Dental Association about infection control guidance and vCJD.* Available from: http://www. dh.gov.uk/en/Publicationsandstatistics/Lettersandcirculars/Dearcolleagueletters/ DH_074431 [accessed 13th March 2010]

Department of Health (2009) *Health Technical Memorandum 01–05: Decontamination in primary care dental practices.* Available from: http://www.dh.gov.uk/en/ Publicationsandstatistics/Publications/PublicationsPolicyAndGuidance/DH_109363 [accessed 13th March 2010]

Medicines Devices Agency (2002) *MAC manual. Part 1: Describing the general principles of the processes that are available for decontamination.* Crown copyright, London

National Institute for Health and Clinical Excellence (NICE) (2006) *Patient safety and reduction of risk of transmission of Creutzfeldt–Jakob disease (CJD) via interventional procedures.* Available from: http://www.nice.org.uk/guidance/index. jsp?action=byID&r=true&o=11332 [accessed 30th May 2010]

NHS Estates (2000) *Decontamination review. Report on a survey of current decontamination practices in healthcare premises in England.* Available from: http://www. dh.gov.uk/en/Publicationsandstatistics/Publications/PublicationsPolicyAndGuidance/ DH_4120917 [accessed 13th March 2010]

NHS Estates (2003a) *A guide to the decontamination of reusable surgical instruments.* Available from: http://www.dh.gov.uk/en/Publicationsandstatistics/Publications/ PublicationsPolicyAndGuidance/DH_4120906 [accessed 13th March 2010]

NHS Estates (2003b) *Decontamination programme. Strategy for modernising the provision of decontamination services.* Available from: http://www.dh.gov.uk/en/ Publicationsandstatistics/Lettersandcirculars/Dearcolleagueletters/DH_4005492 [accessed 13th March 2010]

Perry C (2007) *Infection prevention and control.* Blackwell, Oxford

Glossary

Abnormal prion protein: A form of protein thought to be the causative agent of transmissible spongiform encephalopathies, e.g. CJD. The protein is remarkably resistant to conventional methods of disinfection and sterilisation.

Automated endoscope reprocessor (AER): A machine intended for the decontamination of endoscopes. The AER will have a disinfection phase and may also include a washing phase prior to the disinfection cycle. Many AERs have integrated fume extraction systems.

Bioburden: The population of viable infectious agents contaminating a medical device.

Cleaning: A process which physically removes infectious agents and the organic matter on which they thrive but does not necessarily destroy infectious agents. The reduction of microbial contamination depends upon many factors, including the effectiveness of the cleaning process and the initial bioburden. Cleaning is an essential prerequisite to ensure effective disinfection or sterilisation.

Contamination: The soiling or pollution of inanimate objects or living material with harmful, potentially infectious or other unwanted material. In the clinical situation, this is most likely to be organic matter and infectious agents but may also include other undesirable substances, e.g. chemical residues, radioactive material, degradation products, packaging materials, etc. Such contamination may have an adverse effect on the function of a medical device and may be transferred to a person during use or subsequent processing and storage.

Decontamination: A process that removes or destroys contamination so that infectious agents or other contaminants cannot reach a susceptible site in sufficient quantities to initiate infection or any other harmful response. Differing levels of decontamination are used depending on the device and the procedure involved. The levels of decontamination are either cleaning followed by high level disinfection or cleaning followed by sterilisation.

Disinfectant: A chemical agent which under defined conditions is capable of disinfection.

Disinfection: A process used to reduce the number of viable infectious agents but which may not necessarily inactivate some microbial agents, such as certain viruses and bacterial spores. Disinfection does not achieve the same reduction in microbial contamination levels as sterilisation.

High level disinfectant: A liquid chemical agent which can kill bacteria, viruses and spores. It is only sporicidal under certain conditions.

Infectious agent: The term includes microorganisms and other transmissible agents, e.g. prions.

Single-use: A medical device which is intended to be used on an individual patient during a single procedure and then discarded. It is not intended to be used on another patient.

Sporicide: A chemical agent that, under defined conditions, is capable of killing bacterial spores.

Sterilant: A liquid chemical agent which can kill bacteria, viruses and spores. However this term is not precise and is not commonly used. The term high level disinfectant is preferred.

Sterile Service Department (SSD): A centralised department specifically designed to reprocess re-usable medical devices and equipment and to distribute pre-sterilised, commercially prepared packages for clinical use.

Sterilisation: A process used to render an object free from viable infectious agents including viruses and bacterial spores.

Washer-disinfector: An automated machine intended to clean and disinfect medical devices.

CHAPTER 7

Protective measures

Andrea Denton and Christine Berry

Purpose

The purpose of this chapter is to examine the protective measures required to prevent the transmission of infection. It aims to outline the major principles around standard precautions and provide information and evidence to support the rationale as to why standard precautions are at the centre of infection prevention and control.

Learning outcomes

By the end of the chapter, you will have learned:

- Best practice around hand hygiene.
- Uniform and personal protective equipment.
- Safe management of secretions, blood and body fluids.
- Management of linen.
- Principles of safe waste disposal.

Introduction

Protective measures are used in order to prevent and control the transmission of potentially infectious microorganisms and are more commonly referred to as 'standard precautions' (previously known as universal precautions) (Centre for Disease Control and Prevention 1987). They were originally developed in order to reduce the risk of transmission of blood-borne viruses to healthcare workers. However, not all patients who may be colonised or infected with a pathogenic microorganism or virus are immediately identifiable. Potentially, pathogenic microorganisms no longer just incorporate blood-borne viruses. Therefore, standard precautions are now recommended and should be applied by all healthcare workers at all times when caring for patients.

Knowledge and application of standard infection prevention and control principles within health and social care settings can help to minimise the risks of transmission of potentially infectious microorganisms. Standard precautions encompass hand hygiene, the use of personal, protective equipment (PPE), handling and disposal of sharps, handling and disposal of waste, management of linen, and managing blood and bodily fluids.

Healthcare-associated infections (HCAIs)

An HCAI, previously known as a hospital acquired infection, is one that

...encompasses any infection by any infectious agent acquired as a consequence of a person's treatment by the NHS or which is acquired by a healthcare worker in the course of their NHS duties.

(The Health Act 2006: 1)

The most common HCAIs are urinary tract infections, respiratory tract infections, surgical site infections and blood stream infections (Health Protection Agency 2008a).

Current HCAIs are not a new phenomenon but their profile has risen over the past few years owing to increasing public concern, increased awareness due to improved reporting systems, as well as media coverage and initiatives by the Government to reduce both methicillin-resistant *Staphylococcus aureus* (MRSA) and *Clostridium difficile* rates, in particular (Health Protection Agency 2007).

National Evidence-based Guidelines for Preventing Healthcare-associated Infections in NHS Hospitals in England (EPIC Guidelines) were originally published in 2001 (Pratt et al 2001). They were commissioned by the Department of Health and a revised version was published in 2007 (known as EPIC 2). Both guidelines outline the precautions that should be taken by healthcare workers, focusing upon three main areas: standard principles for the prevention of HCAIs, which includes areas around protective measures; the prevention of infections associated with the use of short-term indwelling urethral catheters; and the prevention of infections related to the use of central venous catheters.

The Health Act (2006) and the subsequent Health and Social Care Act (2008) highlight the importance of embedding the effective prevention and control of HCAIs into day-to-day practice and ensuring that it is applied consistently by all healthcare workers.

Hand hygiene

Effective hand hygiene is one of the most important measures in reducing the spread of infection and one of the fundamental aspects of standard precautions (Gould 1991, Weston 2008). The EPIC 2 Guidelines highlight epidemiological evidence

114

Historical fact

It was an Austrian obstetrician, Semmelweis, who first discovered the link between transmission of organisms and hand contamination. On an obstetric ward where medical students were involved in the care, Semmelweis found that the mortality rate of the patients was over 10% and reached 20% during some months. In contrast, where student midwives received instruction there were very few deaths.

He found that the medical students had attended post mortems prior to entering the ward and examining patients. Semmelweis instigated a vigorous regime of hand scrubbing with soap and water alongside chlorinated lime solution prior to and after examining any patient.

The resulting death rate dropped to less than 1% (Lyons date unknown). Semmelweis is often referred to today in relation to the importance of hand washing and the prevention of cross-infection (National Patient Safety Agency 2004).

---

that suggests that hand-based cross-contamination is a major contributing factor to hospital infection (Pratt et al 2007). However, Pratt et al (2007) do concede that the evidence gained is from quasi-experimental studies, non-randomised trials and expert opinion as opposed to robust randomised-controlled trials. This is due in part to some of the ethical issues and other difficulties in designing and undertaking such studies around hand hygiene compliance.

Resident flora (microorganisms that are present on the hands most of the time) and transient flora (microorganism that are deposited on the hands during healthcare activity and can be transferred to other vulnerable patients) can be cross-transmitted to specific areas, for example surgical wounds, pressure ulcer wounds, intravascular cannula sites, urinary catheter systems and other invasive devices. Therefore it is important that hands are decontaminated at the following times:

- Prior to every episode of care that involves direct contact with patients' skin, food, invasive devices or dressings.
- Following completion of an episode of care and/or after removing gloves.

Pratt et al (2001, 2007)

The 'cleanyourhands' campaign by the National Patient Safety Agency (2004) continues to promote the importance of every individual having a responsibility in the prevention of infection. Areas outside the acute hospital setting are also included as well as the acute sector, with the emphasis of hand hygiene across all environments still very much at the centre of the prevention of HCAIs (Department of Health 2008). Whilst the campaign for the use of alcohol hand rubs has become a feature in this promotion, with hand gel dispensers being seen around all areas, as well as individual healthcare practitioners carrying the portable versions, the emphasis, especially around certain aspects of infection prevention, is good thorough hand washing. Certain bacteria, for example the spores from *Clostridium difficile*, are not destroyed by alcohol alone (Department of Health 2007) and alcohol gel does not remove organic matter.

Five moments for hand hygiene

The five moments for hand hygiene (National Patient Safety Agency 2004) were developed by the World Health Organization (WHO) to identify the critical moments during patient care when staff need to clean their hands in order to prevent the transmission of microorganisms that may cause an HCAI. See *Box 7.1* and *Figure 4.2* on page 64.

Soap and water versus alcohol hand gel

The EPIC 2 guidelines advocate the following:

* Hands that are visibly soiled or potentially grossly contaminated with dirt or organic material (i.e. following the removal of gloves) must be washed with liquid soap and water.
* Hands should be decontaminated between patients or between different care

---

Box 7.1. Five moments for hand hygiene

* Before patient contact
* Before a clean/aseptic procedure
* After body fluid exposure risk
* After patient contact
* After contact with patient's surroundings

Adapted from National Patient Safety Agency (2004)

---

activities for the same patient. This may include using alcohol-based hand rub when appropriate.

- Local infection control guidelines may advise an alternative product to hand rub in some outbreak situations.
- Hands should be washed with soap and water after several consecutive applications of alcohol hand rub.

Hand hygiene technique

There are a variety of visual diagrams to demonstrate techniques for both hand washing and for decontaminating with alcohol hand rub. However the principles are the same and many encompass the stages and important techniques included in *Table 7.1*.

The principles of Stage 2 should be adhered to when applying alcohol-based hand rub.

Issues and barriers around hand hygiene compliance

The issues and barriers around hand hygiene compliance include the following.

- Healthcare staff have a perception that they decontaminate their hands more than they actually do (Harris et al 2000 cited in Wilson 2006).
- Lack of time and facilities, for example hand wash basins to undertake hand hygiene (in particular hand washing).
- Hand washing practice not directly linked to risk of cross-contamination/

Table 7.1. Hand hygiene technique adapted from EPIC 2		
Stage 1: Preparation	*Stage 2: Washing and rinsing*	*Stage 3: Drying*
• Wet hands under running water prior to applying liquid soap/ antimicrobial preparation	• Cover and rub vigorously all surfaces of the hands/wrists paying attention to tips of fingers, backs of hands/fingers, between the fingers, thumbs and wrists • Duration should be a minimum of 10-15 seconds • Rinse thoroughly	• Dry with good quality paper towels

infection. Staff often wash their hands after a low risk activity rather than prior to a high risk activity (Pittet et al 1999).

- Medical staff are especially unlikely to wash their hands (Pittet et al 1999).
- Increasing alcohol hand rub dispensers and feedback to healthcare staff can improve hand hygiene compliance (Brown et al 2003, cited in Pratt et al 2007, Pittet et al 1999).
- Recognising that a multifaceted approach to hand hygiene compliance, including influences on behaviour, can help in a sustained improvement (Pratt et al 2007, Wilson 2006).

Uniform and personal protective equipment

Uniform and workwear

Uniform or work clothing needs to be safe, practical, comfortable and smart, allowing free movement and, amongst other things, should project a positive image to patients and clients (Royal College of Nursing 2009). However, whilst the main objective of a uniform is to project a corporate image, uniform also has a function under the Health and Safety at Work Act (1974), which is to protect staff and patients. Under the Health and Social Care Act (2008), in order to minimise the risk of HCAIs, uniforms should be clean and fit for purpose.

Although there is no conclusive evidence that uniforms have any impact on spreading infection (Department of Health 2010), work clothes may become contaminated by bacteria (Royal College of Nursing 2009). Therefore it is important that the clothes worn by healthcare workers should minimise risk to patients. Any workwear or uniform should facilitate good hand hygiene compliance and not come into direct contact with patients during any patient care activity.

The Department of Health guidance on uniform and workwear (2010) outlines the main principles. The guidance maintains that much of the uniform and workwear advice is based on good practice and requires 'no evidence base' but is based on safety, comfort and public confidence (Department of Health 2010). Adapted below are some of these guidelines in relation to infection prevention and control with other evidence sourced and referenced where appropriate (see *Table 7.2*).

Personal protective equipment (PPE)

PPE refers to gloves, aprons, masks, eye protection, hats and footwear which protect staff and patients from infections or hazardous products. PPE is used to

Table 7.2. Guidelines for uniform	
• Supply and laundering uniforms and workwear	• Staff should have sufficient uniforms to enable a clean uniform every day • There is little evidence to suggest that there is any difference between domestic and commercial laundering • A 10-minute wash at 60°C removes all microorganisms. Any contaminated uniforms should be changed immediately (Department of Health 2010)
• Changing into and out of uniform at work/covering uniform completely if travelling to and from work • Engage in activities outside work in uniform	• There is no evidence of infection risk when travelling in uniform but public perception is that it is unhygienic (Department of Health 2010) • There is no evidence of infection risk but public perception perceives there to be a risk
• Bare below the elbow	• Jewellery and watches can harbour microorganisms and make effective hand hygiene more problematic (Salisbury et al 1997) • Local policy may allow a plain wedding band
• Clean, short, unvarnished fingernails (including non-false nails)	• Long nails harbour more microorganisms and pierce gloves (Provincial Infectious Diseases Advisory Committee 2007)

reduce the potential exposure to infective agents and materials and thus reduces the potential spread to other patients and staff (Clark et al 2002). Selecting PPE should be based on a risk assessment of the patient, the environment and the risk of transmitting pathogens. Health and safety regulations, including Personal Protective Equipment at Work Regulations 1992 alongside Control of Substances Hazardous to Health (COSHH) regulations (2002), provide clear guidance and direction for employers ensuring that PPE is available and appropriate and that staff have been trained in its proper use (Hinkin et al 2008).

Pratt et al (2007) highlight in the EPIC 2 guidelines that there is evidence to suggest a lack of knowledge and poor adherence to PPE use and maintain that more education around risk assessment and correct use is required. The principles for selection and use of PPE are outlined below.

Gloves

- Pratt et al (2007) highlight the importance of correct use and risk assessment when determining if gloves are required and the selection of the most appropriate type and material in order to avoid adverse reactions.
- Gloves should be worn whenever there may be direct contact with mucous membranes, body fluids, broken skin and during invasive procedures and contact with sterile sites. Gloves provide a reliable method for reducing the number of microorganisms on hands (Pittet et al 1999).
- Gloves should be applied immediately before patient contact and removed immediately following contact. It is important to change gloves (and decontaminate hands) between different patients, or between different procedures for the same patient (Wilson 2006).
- Gloves are not a substitute for hand washing.
- Hands should be decontaminated before and after using gloves (Health Protection Agency 2009).
- Gloves are single-use items and should be disposed of as clinical waste (Health Protection Scotland 2010).
- Gloves should conform to European Community (CE) standards and must not be powdered or made from polythene. Alternatives to natural rubber latex gloves should be available for use in case of latex allergy.
- Avoid prolonged and indiscriminate use of gloves.

Aprons

- Disposable aprons should be worn when there is a risk that clothing may be exposed or contaminated with blood and/or body fluids and if there is direct contact with infectious patients or clients and their environment.
- They should be single use and disposed of after use as clinical waste or domestic waste depending on the activity and the patient's infection risk (Health Protection Scotland 2010).
- Hands should be decontaminated prior to putting on aprons and if an apron is used for specific single patient use it should be changed between patients.

- Full body fluid-repellent gowns should be used when the risk of contamination is likely to be extensive (Health Protection Scotland 2010).

Face masks and visors/eye protection

- There are a variety of face masks including ordinary surgical face masks, particulate filter masks and FFP3 particulate filter respirators; the latter requiring a 'fit test' prior to being used.
  - Particulate filter masks are clinically indicated when infection is spread by the airborne route. They should be properly fitted and handled as little as possible. These are used for patients with or suspected of having pulmonary TB in the first 2 weeks of treatment and should be used for aerosol-generating procedures only (see *Box 7.2* for examples of aerosol-generating procedures).
  - FFP3 masks should be worn when indicated by infection prevention and control teams but instances may include multidrug resistant TB (MDRTB) (NICE 2006) and severe respiratory syndrome (SARS) (Pratt et al 2007). FFP3 masks were also indicated for aerosol generating procedures in the 2009 H1N1 pandemic influenza outbreak (swine flu) (Health Protection Scotland 2009).
- Eye/face protection should be worn if there is a risk of blood or body fluids splashing into the face. This can be in the form of goggles or visors depending on the nature of the patient episode/contact.

Box 7.2. Aerosol-generating procedures

- Dry cough-inducing procedures
- Chest physiotherapy
- Nebulisers
- Suctioning
- Inhalation and pentamidine medication
- Bronchoscopy
- During prolonged care of a high dependant patient

NICE (2006)

Management of secretions, blood and body fluids

Any blood and body fluids, including secretions (see *Box 7.3*), must be managed using the principles of standard precautions. It is important to assume that any secretions/body fluids are a potential risk of infection and therefore good hand hygiene, effective and efficient use of PPE, and effective cleaning of the environment and equipment should be adopted (Wilson 2006, Kilpatrick et al 2008).

Box 7.3. Examples of body fluids/secretions

• Saliva	• Sputum	• Faeces
• Breast milk	• Blood	• Urine
• Vomit	• Semen	• Vaginal secretions
• Sweat	• Tears	• Droplets from coughing, sneezing

Spillages

Spillages need to be dealt with effectively and efficiently according to the workplace's written policy. Policies should include information regarding the nature of the chemical to be used to ensure that the spillage is safely disinfected and to ensure an appropriate solution is used where the spillage occurred, for example a carpet in a patient's home (Royal College of Nursing 2004). Any action should be undertaken in a prompt and timely manner.

Collection, handling and labelling of specimens

All specimens should be collected appropriately and in the most effective sterile container to ensure safe collection and transportation and to minimise risk to both the collector and laboratory staff. Safe transportation of specimens needs to comply with COSHH regulations (2002) and the Health and Safety at Work Act (1974), and workplace policies need to reflect this.

Isolation precautions

In certain circumstances where there is a risk of infection, isolation procedures may also need to be applied in order to help to reduce further the risk of cross-contamination. All these aspects are more applicable in healthcare institutions, such as hospitals, but may also be applicable and adapted to care home facilities (Nazarko 2007). The principles of isolation precautions began in hospitals in the early 20th century but have been around generally since biblical times. There was a growing recognition that infection was often spread from person to person and precautions including 'barrier precautions' could be effective in reducing transmission.

Although the initial concept of universal (standard) precautions was concerned with the reduction of transmission of blood-borne viruses and was introduced at the time of growing concerns around HIV, the change in emphasis to all blood and bodily fluids being a potential major source of infection and cross-transmission has had major implications for isolation precautions (Wilson 2006). Today there are a variety of isolation precautions and different definitions depending on the workplace. The decision to isolate depends on assessment and the risk of dispersal of the known or suspected infectious microorganism to other vulnerable patients and healthcare staff, as well as to the patient's condition (Kilpatrick et al 2008).

There are a variety of different types of isolation precautions; the most common one is a single room with en suite facilities. Other isolation precautions include rooms with controlled ventilation for airborne or respiratory risks. The type and nature of isolation depends on the patient, environment of care and reason for isolation; the overall aim is to reduce the risk of transmission. Discussion with the infection prevention and control team can help in deciding on the most appropriate type. Isolation needs to be undertaken in conjunction with other standard precautions (Kilpatrick et al 2008).

Management of sharps/accidental exposure to body fluids

Safe handling and disposal of needles and other sharps continues to be one of the main concerns around injuries to NHS staff, secondary only to moving and handling injuries (National Audit office 2003). In a recent report by the Health Protection Agency (2008b) there were 914 incidents between 2006 and 2007 where healthcare workers were put at risk. Between 2000 and 2007, 48% of incidents involved nurses. Procedures for the safe handling of sharps are shown in *Box 7.4*.

The main area of concern is around exposure to blood-borne viruses, namely HIV, hepatitis B and hepatitis C. Exposure can occur via the following routes:

• Percutaneous injury (needles, instruments, bites that break the skin).

Box 7.4. Safe handling of sharps

- Avoid direct handling of needles
- Never re-sheath, break or bend needles
- Never pass sharps to another person directly
- If possible, use needleless cannulae
- Always enlist help if using sharps near a confused or restless patient
- Always dispose of sharp and carrier device as a single unit
- Always place used needles and blades directly into an approved sharps container at point of use
- Fill sharps containers only to three quarters capacity then seal and label
- Always ensure temporary closure mechanism is in place on all sharps containers when not in use
- Know your organisation's sharps policies

Adapted from Hardy (2009)

- Exposure via broken skin (abrasions, cuts, skin conditions such as eczema).
- Exposure of mucous membranes (including eyes and mouth).

Post-exposure prophylaxis (PEP) for HIV, vaccination for hepatitis B (HBV) and post-exposure follow up tests for hepatitis C (HCV) are vital to help reduce the number of seroconversion cases. To date (data available from 1997–2007) the number of HCV seroconversions in healthcare workers in England is 14 and HIV in the UK is five (Health Protection Agency 2008b). The report by the HPA highlighted a major concern in the lack of testing and follow up of HCV and emphasis is placed on the healthcare worker understanding that infection can go undetected for many years. There is also mention of the fact that many of the injuries sustained, especially around percutaneous injuries, were preventable.

Comprehensive workplace and occupational health policies are required to ensure that risks are minimised and the management of any injury related to blood-borne virus exposure is robust and timely.

Managing injuries/accidents

For an example of how to manage any blood-borne virus exposure see *Box 7.5*. Also, always refer to workplace/trust policy guidelines. In line with the Health

---

Box 7.5. Management of blood-borne virus exposure

- Immediately stop what you are doing and attend injury
- Encourage bleeding (apply gentle pressure)
- Wash under running water
- If body fluids splash into eyes irrigate with cold water. If body fluids splash into mouth do not swallow, rinse out several times with cold water
- Report incident to occupational health or A & E out of hours department
- Inform manager
- Complete accident/incident form
- In case of injury from clean/unused instrument or needle no further action is necessary
- In case of a used needle or instrument, risk assessment should be carried out and discussed with microbiologist, infection prevention and control doctor, or consultant for communicable disease
- Seek help to investigate cause and risk assessment

Adapted from Royal College of Nursing (2004)

---

and Safety at Work Act 1984, all workplaces should display posters and/or visible information regarding management of blood-borne virus exposure.

Management of linen

The management of linen is an important aspect of infection prevention and control. Non-compliance with recommended practice can contribute to the spread of potentially harmful microorganisms within the environment and between patients, staff and/or residents.

> *The NHS has an obligation under the Health and Safety at Work Act to take steps to prevent the risk of infection to staff handling and laundering linen.*
>
> (NHS Executive 1995)

There is also legislation relating to the Registered Homes Act in respect of laundry from small units, with which managers are expected to comply. Laundry/management of linen policies should be available in all care settings regarding appropriate handling of clean or used linen. Guidance exists to promote safe practice, to reduce the risk of infection to staff, and to ensure appropriate decontamination of used and infected linen.

All staff handling linen should receive appropriate training to carry out their duties efficiently and safely (NHS Executive 1995).

Laundry requirements in care settings consist of:

- Adequate supply of clean linen.
- Appropriately coloured linen bags.
- Water soluble bags.
- Laundering facilities that meet the required standards in order to ensure the appropriate disinfection of used linen, i.e. machines that are able to achieve temperatures of 65°C for 10 minutes or 71°C for 3 minutes.
- Clean, dry, storage area (not in a sluice, dirty utility room or bathroom).

All NHS trusts are asked to work towards implementing the national colour standard (see *Table 7.3*). All laundry should be segregated in order that users and those managing or processing laundry understand what type of laundry is in each bag and how to process and clean specific laundry (NHS Executive 1995). See *Table 7.4* for categories for used laundry.

Table 7.3. National colour standard for linen

Used linen	*White or off-white container*
Infected linen	Red container or red as a prominent feature on a white or off-white background
Heat labile linen	White with a prominent orange stripe

Table 7.4. Categories for used laundry

Special laundry	Items that may be damaged in a hot wash such as woollens or patients'/ residents' own clothing
Fouled/infected linen	Laundry contaminated with blood or body fluids or used by patients with known infections such as MRSA or who have infestations such as fleas
Used laundry	Used laundry not contaminated with blood or body fluids
Theatre linen	Linen generated from theatre settings; green bags are usually used

Curtains

Curtains used within ward areas or other care settings should be on an agreed programme for regular changing and they should be changed if visibly soiled. They should also be changed if an area requires a terminal clean, for example following an outbreak of viral gastroenteritis.

Use of washing machines in ward areas

- This should not occur without prior agreement between the ward manager, the infection prevention and control team and the estates/facilities department. Domestic appliances are not suitable.
- If ward-based laundry facilities are available, these must not be situated within a clinical area.
- A hand wash basin that is easily accessible should be available.
- There should be a separate area for drying and ironing clean laundry.

A summary of the main points to remember when handling used linen are shown in *Table 7.5.*

Table 7.5. Rules for handling used linen	
Do	Don't
• Handle used laundry with care	• Shake, waft or throw
• Always use a linen skip, if available	used laundry
• Place used linen into the appropriate linen bag at the point of use	• Place on inappropriate surfaces, such as the
• Wear appropriate PPE, i.e. a disposable apron	floor or a table
• Disposable gloves should be worn for handling fouled/infected laundry	• Walk through a ward or other areas carrying
• Use the appropriate-coloured linen bag	used linen
• Use a water-soluble bag to dispose of linen used by a patient with an infection	• Overfill laundry bags; they should not be
• Remove used laundry to an appropriate holding area; do not leave in the same area as a patient or resident, e.g. a side-room or bedroom	more than three-quarters full
• Ensure that there are no inappropriate items mixed up in used laundry	• Store linen bags/skips in side rooms/bedrooms

Disposal of waste

It is estimated that the NHS produces approximately 250 000 tonnes of waste each year, disposed of in landfill sites or by incineration. The NHS has a legal duty to dispose of waste in accordance with the duty of care requirements imposed under the Environmental Protection Act (1990, Section 34) and the Environmental Protection (Duty of Care) Regulations 1991 (Department of Health 2009).

The Health Technical Memorandum (HTM 070-01) (Department of Health 2006) recommends that all health and social care settings should have an up-to-date waste management policy outlining the role and responsibilities of all concerned with the segregation and disposal of waste. This memorandum, produced by the Department of Health, contains guidance relating to best practice for the storage, carriage, treatment and disposal of waste. There are many regulations governing waste disposal; a detailed list can be found within the document itself, which can be downloaded from the Department of Health website.

The European Commission produces a European Waste Catalogue in accordance with the European Waste Framework Directive in order to provide common terminology for describing waste throughout Europe.

Healthcare waste

Healthcare waste refers to any waste produced by and as a consequence of healthcare activities.

(Department of Health 2006: 7)

Guidance on the safe disposal of healthcare waste also applies to offensive/ hygiene and infectious waste produced in the community from non-NHS healthcare sources.

Segregation of waste

Segregation of waste is a common issue raised in health and social care settings and it is important to identify the correct waste stream for the disposal of various items. It is recommended that all staff should be provided with clear instructions on the segregation process and receive the appropriate training. In order to assist with this process, colour-coded waste receptacles should be supplied for each waste stream.

The main types of waste within health and social care settings, unless in a specialised area, are: domestic waste, offensive waste, hazardous/infectious waste, medicinal waste, cytotoxic and cytostatic waste, and waste electrical and electronic equipment (WEEE). *Table 7.6* provides a summary of the types of waste stream and definitions.

Table 7.6. Waste streams

Waste stream	Definition
Anatomical waste	• Body parts or other recognisable anatomical items
Domestic waste	• The same as, or similar to, waste generated from the home and not containing any infectious material or sharps
Medicinal waste (other than cytotoxic/ cytostatic)	• Expired, unused, spilt and contaminated pharmaceutical products, drugs, vaccines and sera that are no longer required. Includes packaging that may be contaminated with residues, gloves, masks, connecting tubing, syringe bodies and drug vials
Infectious/ hazardous waste	• Substances containing viable microorganisms or their toxins, which are known, or reliably believed, to cause disease in man or living organisms
Offensive/ hygiene waste	• Waste that may cause offence due to the presence of recognisable healthcare waste items or body fluids • Does not meet the definition of infectious waste • Does not possess any hazardous properties • Not identified as needing disinfection or any other treatment to reduce the number of microorganisms present
Clinical waste	• Waste that poses a risk of infection
Cytotoxic/ cytostatic waste	• Classified as hazardous waste • A medicinal product possessing one or more of the hazardous properties: toxic, carcinogenic, toxic for reproduction, mutagenic
Sharps waste	• Items that could cause injury, for example cuts and puncture wounds. These include needles, syringes with needles attached, broken glass ampoules, scalpels and other blades and infusion sets (sharp part)
WEEE	• Waste electrical and electronic equipment
	From: HM Government (2005), Department of Health (2006)

It is important that each healthcare worker is aware of and complies with appropriate segregation and disposal of waste. There is a legal requirement as well as moral and ethical issues involved in appropriate waste disposal. It should be remembered that 'all waste has the potential to pollute land, air or water' (Department of Health 2009).

Summary

This chapter has looked at best practice around hand hygiene, standard precautions, and the management of linen and potentially hazardous waste. It has provided an overall outline with some supporting evidence and rationale. Whilst some areas, such as hand hygiene, are well supported with an evidence base; others, for example, uniform wear, tend to be guided by 'best practice' as the Department of Health outlines in its guidelines (Department of Health 2010). The chapter has also provided some of the essential aspects around infection prevention and control that can be utilised across a wide range of care settings, in order to try and reduce the risk of transmission of microorganisms and help to prevent infections. However, it is important to appreciate that hand

---

Reflective exercise

Thinking about all of the different protective measures discussed, i.e. hand hygiene, uniform and personal protective equipment, management of secretions and blood-borne viruses, sharps management, linen and waste:

• Which areas do you consider are undertaken well in your current area of practice?
• Which areas would you consider to be the most challenging concerns in your current area of practice
  • For you
  • For the immediate team you work with
  • For other members of the healthcare team that impact on your everyday work?
• What can you do about any concerns?
• Who else might you involve?
• What can you do to help further your knowledge and understanding around protective measures?

---

hygiene, standard precautions and the safe management of linen and waste are vast areas and as such this chapter has provided just an insight into some of the main principles.

In the next chapter we will look specifically at the protective measures required when handling food and water supplies including potable water and ice.

References

Brown SM, Lubimova AV, Khrustalyeva NM, et al (2003) Use of an alcohol-based hand rub and quality improvement interventions to improve hand hygiene in a Russian neonatal intensive care unit. *Infection Control and Hospital Epidemiology* 24: 172–9

Centre for Disease Control and Prevention (1987) *Universal precautions*. Available from: http://www.cdc.gov/ncidod/dhqp/bp_universal_precautions.html [Accessed 25 April 2010]

Clark L, Smith W, Young L (2002) *Protective clothing; Principles and guidance*. Infection Control Nurses Association, London

Department of Health (2006) *Health Technical Memorandum 07-01: Safe management of healthcare waste*. Department of Health, London

Department of Health (2007) *A simple guide to clostridium difficile*. Available from: http://www.dh.gov.uk/en/Publichealth/Healthprotection/Healthcareacquiredinfection/ Healthcareacquiredgeneralinformation/DH_4115800 [Accessed 11 April 2010

Department of Health (2008) *Changes to arrangements for regulating NHS bodies in relation to healthcare associated infections for 2009/10. A consultation document*. Department of Health, London

Department of Health (2009) *Waste*. Available from: http://www.dh.gov.uk/en/ Managingyourorganisation/Estatesandfacilitiesmanagement/Sustainabledevelopment/ DH_4119635 [Accessed 23 March 2010]

Department of Health (2010) *Uniforms and workwear: Guidance on uniform and workwear policies for NHS employers*. Department of Health, London

Gould D (1991) Nurses' hands as vectors of hospital acquired infections: A review. *Journal of Advanced Nursing* 16: 1216–25

Hardy J (2009) Learning the hard way. *Nursing Standard* 23(35): 61

Health and Safety Executive (1992) *Personal Protective Equipment at Work Regulations: Guidance on Regulations*. Health and Safety Executive, London. Available from: http://www.hse.gov.uk/pubns/indg174.pdf

Health Protection Agency (2007) *The surveillance of healthcare associated infections report 2007*. Health Protection Agency, London

Health Protection Agency (2008a) *The surveillance of HCAIs report*. Health Protection Agency, London

Health Protection Agency (2008b) *Eye of the needle*. Health Protection Agency, London

Health Protection Agency (2009) *Pandemic (H1N1) 2009 Influenza: information for health professionals*. Available from: http://www.hpa.org.uk/Topics/InfectiousDiseases/ InfectionsAZ/SwineInfluenza/SIProfessional/ [Accessed June 23 2010]

Health Protection Scotland (2010) *Personal protective equipment sources*. Available from: http://www.hps.scot.nhs.uk/haiic/ic/publicationsdetail.aspx?id=33886 [Accessed 8 August 2010]

Hinkin J, Gammon J, Cutter J (2008) *Review of personal protection equipment used in practice*. British Journal of Community Nursing **13**(3): 14–19

HM Government (2005) *Hazardous waste regulations*. HM Government, London

Kilpatrick C, Prieto J, Wigglesworth N (2008) Single room isolation to prevent the transmission of infection: Development of a patient journey tool to support safe practice. *Journal of Hospital Infection* **9**(6): 19–25

Lyons AS (date unknown) *Medical history - Infection*. Available from: http://www.health-guidance.org/entry/6354/1/Medical-History--Infection.html [Accessed 22 March 2010]

Nazarko L (2007) *Standard precautions in infection control*. Nursing and Residential Care **9**(10): 463–6

National Audit Office (2003) *A safer place to work: Improving the management of health and safety risks to staff in NHS Trusts*. National Audit office, London

National Institute for Health and Clinical Excellence (2006) *Tuberculosis: Clinical diagnosis and management of tuberculosis and measures for its prevention and control*. National Institute for Health and Clinical Excellence, London

National Patient Safety Agency (2004) *Cleanyourhands (CYH) campaign*. National Patient Safety Agency, London

NHS Executive (1995) *Hospital laundry arrangements for used and infected linen*. HSG 95 (18). NHS Executive., London

Pittet D, Dharan S, Touveneau S, Sauvan V, Perneger T (1999) Bacterial contamination of the hands of hospital staff during routine patient care. *Archives of Internal Medicine* **159**: 821–6

Pratt RJ, Pellowe C, Loveday HP, et al (2001) The Epic Project: Developing national evidence-based guidelines for preventing healthcare associated infections. Phase 1: Guidelines for preventing hospital-acquired infections. *Journal of Hospital Infection*

47(Supplement): S1–S82

Pratt RJ, Pellowe CM, Wilson JA, et al. (2007). Epic 2: National evidence-based guidelines for preventing healthcare-associated infections in NHS hospitals in England. *Journal of Hospital Infection* **65S**: S1–S64

Provincial Infectious Diseases Advisory Committee (2007) *Hand Hygiene. Fact Sheet for health care settings*. Available from: http://www.health.gov.on.ca/english/providors/program/infectious/diseases/best _prac/bp_hh_20080501.pdf [Accessed 14 April 2010]

Royal College of Nursing (2004) *Good practice in infection control*. Royal College of Nursing, London

Royal College of Nursing (2009) *Guidance on uniforms and work wear*. Royal College of Nursing, London

Salisbury DM, Hutfilz P, Treen LM, Solin GE, Gautam S (1997) The effect of rings on microbial load of health care workers' hands. *American Journal of Infection Control* 25: 24–7

Weston D (2008) *Infection prevention and control*. John Wiley & Sons Ltd, London

Wilson J (2006) *Infection control in clinical practice* (3rd edn). Balliere Tindall, London

Useful Websites

Care Quality Commission: http://www.cqc.org.uk/

Department of Health: http://www.dh.gov.uk/en/Home

Health Protection Agency: http://www.hpa.org.uk/

National Patient Safety Agency: http://www.npsa.nhs.uk/

National Institute for Health and Clinical Excellence: http://www.nice.org.uk/

Royal College of Nursing: http://www.rcn.org.uk/

CHAPTER 8

Special precautions

Carole Hallam and Sandra Mogford

Purpose

This chapter covers some of the control measures needed to provide safe food and water within the healthcare setting. It also looks at some of the main infections related to both elements.

Learning outcome

By the end of the chapter, you will have learned:

- The key food and water-borne infections.
- The four components to good food hygiene.
- The principles of safe handling of potable water.
- Best practice to prevent water-borne infections.

Introduction

A number of significant outbreaks of food-borne illness and food poisoning in healthcare settings have occurred over the past 15 years, affecting both acute hospitals and nursing homes. Wall et al (1996) reviewed 22 hospital outbreaks of food-borne illness and concluded that of the 22 outbreaks in which *Salmonella* spp. were implicated, person-to-person spread accounted for 12, food-borne infection for eight and the route of infection was unknown in the other two.

Food-borne outbreaks are also reported from nursing homes; two outbreaks were reported to the Health Protection Agency in 2009, one from *Clostridium perfringens* affecting 28 residents and the second affecting eight residents where *Salmonella enteritidis* was isolated (Health Protection Agency 2010a).

Food hygiene requirements for businesses are made under statutory regulations given by the Food Safety Act 1990. The Act is a wide-ranging legislation on food safety and consumer protection in relation to food and includes non-profit making organisations, including the NHS. Local policies and guidelines for food hygiene should be available and staff performing food handling duties should be appropriately trained (Department of Health 2009a).

Hygiene is not only to be considered in terms of food handling but also in the handling and management of water and water supplies. Of all the potential water-borne infections, legionnaires' disease is probably the most serious, with 12% of cases of legionellosis being fatal. *Legionella* was first recognised in 1976 following an outbreak of infection amongst people attending an American Legion Convention. Between 1980 and 2008, there was a total of 233 confirmed cases of legionnaires' disease attributed to hospitals, of these, 151 were part of an outbreak (Health Protection Agency 2010b) and the rest were isolated cases.

To some extent the principles around managing food can be applied to safe handling of water and water systems. We will begin by looking more closely at safe food handling.

The four 'C's of good food hygiene

There are four main components to good food hygiene, often referred to as the four 'C's (Food Standards Agency 2005).

- Cross-contamination.
- Cleaning.
- Chilling.
- Cooking.

Cross-contamination

Healthcare workers involved with the preparation, cooking or serving of food should not only understand basic food hygiene but also realise the added risks in a healthcare setting. With staff working in an environment where pathogenic organisms from faecal matter can potentially contaminate healthcare workers' hands, uniforms and the environment, the risks of cross-contamination to food is high. This presents risks to all patients, and those whose immune systems are compromised due to age, disease and medical treatment are highly susceptible to infection.

Preventing cross-contamination can be achieved with good hand hygiene prior to entering the kitchen area and prior to preparing or serving food. To achieve effective hand hygiene nails should be kept short and nail varnish, wrist jewellery and stoned rings should not be worn (Food Standards Agency 2005, Pratt et al 2007).

The National Patient Safety Agency and the World Health Organization have excellent documentation, including posters, showing correct hand washing techniques using alcohol gel or soap and water (WHO 2006, National Patient Safety Agency 2007). This information can easily be obtained via the internet and most infection prevention and control teams will have the posters or information in their departments. Further information on hand hygiene can be found in *Chapter 7*.

A clean apron should be worn when preparing and/or serving food; these are usually disposable (Food Standards Agency 2005). The benefit of colour coding the apron is to be able to differentiate between a personal hygiene task and a food hygiene task.

Cloths can be one of the top causes of cross-contamination as bacteria thrive in the moist material. Single use cloths, which are thrown away after each task, will negate this risk (Food Standards Agency 2005).

Separating foods to prevent cross-contamination between raw and ready-to-eat food is essential. Where possible, raw food should be stored in a separate fridge (Food Standards Agency 2005). Within the healthcare setting there are potential risks of contamination from food brought in by staff or relatives and stored in fridges along with patients' food. Hospitals and care homes should have local policies and guidelines (Department of Health 2009a) and these should address this risk, but in the absence of local guidance the situation must be carefully assessed and managed and, at the least, this food should be dated and suitably wrapped.

Food handlers, including those who serve food, should be 'fit for work' and not suffering from a communicable disease which could contaminate the food. Healthcare workers and food handlers should not come to work if they have or have had symptoms of diarrhoea and/or vomiting in the last 48 hours. They should remain off work until they have been symptom free for 48 hours (Food Standards Agency 2005).

Box 8.1. Key points to prevent cross-contamination

- Good hand hygiene
- Clean apron
- Single use cloths
- Ready-to-eat food kept separately from raw food
- Do not work with symptoms of diarrhoea or vomiting

Cleaning

Cleaning schedules that identify what should be cleaned, how cleaning should be done, its frequency and who should do it must be available. However, the 'clean as you go' principle should be applied to prevent an accumulation of food debris and unwashed cups left in the sink (Food Standards Agency 2005).

Chilling

Certain foods need to be kept chilled to keep them safe. These include food with a 'use by date'; ready-to-eat foods, such as yoghurts; food that has been cooked but is not to be served straight away; and other food that states it needs to be refrigerated on the label (Food Standards Agency 2005). Within an establishment, it is deemed an offence by the Environmental Health Officers enforcing the Food Safety Law, to store food beyond its 'use by' date alongside food to be consumed by others (Food Standards Agency 1990). Daily checking of the use by dates of food is essential, ensuring that out-of-date food is discarded.

Chilled foods must be kept at 8°C or below. To achieve this, it is recommended that fridges are set at 5°C or below. Temperature of fridges and freezers should be taken and recorded daily. Food that needs to be frozen should be placed in the freezer as soon as it is delivered. Frozen food that has started to thaw should not be returned to the freezer (Food Standards Agency 2005).

Box 8.2. Key points for chilled food

- Do not store or use chilled food after its 'use by' date
- Check and record fridge and freezer temperatures
- Ensure temperature is between 0°–5°C or below
- Report temperatures above 5°C

Cooking

Although most healthcare staff would not be directly involved with cooking food there may be occasions when cooking is required, perhaps associated with assisting or advising patients who are undergoing rehabilitation on cooking food after their discharge (Food Standards Agency 2005). Food should be cooked thoroughly and be piping hot. Food should reach temperatures in excess of 63°C during cooking to kill off harmful bacteria, and then be served as soon as possible. Keeping food warm should be avoided but where there are no alternatives then it should be kept at a minimum of 63°C for no longer than 2 hours, after which time it should be consumed or discarded. Food should not be reheated (Food Standards Agency 2005).

Microwaves are often discouraged in hospital ward kitchens due to the risk of them being used to reheat food for patients. As the heat is not evenly distributed in microwaved food, there is as increased risk that any bacteria present will not be killed off, which may result in food poisoning.

Bacteria thrive in temperatures between 8°C and 60°C and this is often referred to as the 'danger zone'. Keeping food either below or above the danger zone prevents the multiplication of bacteria and thus keeps food safe (Food Standards Agency 2005).

Box 8.3. Key points for cooked food

- Do not reheat food
- Ensure food is above 63°C and piping hot
- Be careful when serving hot food to patients to prevent burns
- Serve promptly

Pest control

Food-borne bacteria can be spread by pests, such as rodents, flies, cockroaches and other crawling insects. Healthcare workers should be vigilant for the presence of pests and any signs should be reported to the pest contractor, or local policy should be followed (Food Standards Agency 2005). Cockroaches have been found to harbour pathogenic bacteria; a study in Taiwan found that nearly all the cockroaches in the hospitals investigated were harbouring bacteria, such as *Staphylococcus aureus, Pseudomonas aerinosa, Serratia marcescens, Klebsiella pneumoniae, Enterococcus* spp. and *Proteus* spp. and most of these were multi-resistant strains (Pai et al 2004). In a neonatal unit in South Africa, Cotton et al

(2000) isolated *Klebsiella pneumoniae* from cockroaches. The *Klebsiella* were indistinguishable from the same organism colonising and causing clinical disease in the babies.

Stop, check, ask...

Do you handle, prepare or serve food to patients in your workplace, if so:
• Are you aware of where the food hygiene policy is kept?
• Have you been trained in food hygiene?
• If you observed a cockroach or similar pest in the kitchen, what would you do?
• If three patients were observed to have symptoms of diarrhoea, what actions will you take according to your local policies?

Water coolers and ice makers

Potable water in the healthcare setting, whether delivered via tap, water cooler or ice maker, is generally accepted to be safe for human consumption. Ayliffe et al (1999) discuss the merits of tap water:

> *Freshly drawn mains water is usually of good microbiological quality and contains very few bacteria ...Heating water dechlorinates it and water standing in tanks or unused lengths of pipework or trapped around tap washers may produce an increase in bacterial counts. Despite these problems tap water is very rarely an infection risk to the healthy person.*

However, there is research that highlights contamination found within some ice makers notably by *Legionella* spp. (Stout et al 1985, Bangsborg et al 1995, Graman et al 1997, Schuetz et al 2009) and *Mycobacterium fortuitum* (Laussucq et al 1988, Gebo et al 2002).

Water coolers

Many healthcare settings have stand-alone water coolers that utilise replaceable water bottles from commercial companies. Points to consider are:

• Is the water of an acceptable quality for susceptible or immunocompromised patients or is it only for the consumption of healthy people, e.g. members of staff?

• Have the water bottles been stored and transported correctly from manufacturer to intended delivery points?

• What happens to the empty bottles: Are they recycled and/or reused?

• How easy is it to remove the protective foil from the bottle and insert the bottle into the machine without environmental contamination?

These water bottles require large storage areas away from strong smells and out of direct sunlight. Some settings use bottle cradles next to the water cooler. If you have ever attempted to replace an empty bottle with a full one you will be only too aware of how difficult it is to manipulate the new bottle into position without the possibility of causing personal body injury.

Whilst these commercial water bottles are manufactured under strict conditions some companies only show a manufacturer's date and/or a consume by date on the bottle label/bottle neck. There does not appear to be any instruction on the timescale of how long the water is safe to be drunk once the bottle is inserted into the machine. In those instances it would be prudent to contact the manufacturers to establish directions for the safe consumption of their water. However, there is no reason why a date should not be put on the bottle label to

---

Activity

In order to provide safe handling of potable water, please access and read the following documents and record any reference made to potable water:

• Healthcare setting policies
• Infection prevention and control policies/guidelines
• Manual handling guidelines
• Available manufacturers' guidelines/recommendations

Now answer the following questions:

• When changing the water bottle, what do the manufacturer's instructions state?
• Does the required task allow you to follow workplace guidelines and policies?
• How can you reduce risks to yourself and others?

clarify when the bottle was inserted into the cooler. It is worth noting that once a bottle of water, of the type bought from a supermarket or grocery store, is opened it should be refrigerated and consumed within four days.

Ice makers

Many people are unaware that the Food Safety Act 1990 identifies water, and therefore ice, as food. The Act requires the handling of food and any contact material, such as ice-making machines, to meet recognised safety standards (Gallagher 1999).

Wilson et al (1997) state that

Hospital outbreaks and recurring infections have sometimes been traced to inadequately maintained ice-making machines.

There could be a lack of knowledge by staff about such equipment needing to be on a maintenance programme or a lack of role definition on cleaning and maintenance of the machines.

Research has shown that if bacterial filters are used, both in the mains supply and machines, there is a reduction of pathogens and therefore nosocomial infections (i.e. infection acquired as a result of treatment within the hospital or healthcare environment) (Bangsborg et al 1995, Wilson et al 1997, Hall et al 2004, Department of Health 2009b).

Following on from these investigations, Gebo et al (2002) suggest that besides increased cleansing (to ice makers),

The use of filters with reduced pore size may actually prevent contamination that may lead to outbreaks [and the] use of filters (particularly in places where biofilms are likely to develop, such as in ice machines) should be considered on a biannual basis.

Filters are not the only effective measure. To reduce nosocomial infections it has been suggested that oxidising agents or ionisation to hospital water supplies can be used (Department of Health 2009b). Clearly these sorts of measures are outside the scope of ward/department healthcare workers.

The importance of hand hygiene in reducing infection can never be over-emphasised and hands should be washed immediately prior to accessing the ice machine. Also, maintaining clear concise records in the cleaning and maintenance of the machine, and reporting faults immediately, will all help towards better functioning.

The ice storage compartment needs to be well insulated, otherwise ice will not be maintained at the correct temperature and may result in melting, especially during hot weather. This collection of water could be a source for water-borne pathogens to survive and accumulate.

Manufacturers should also have a responsibility, indeed it is in their favour, to ensure their machines are of a standard that complies with requirements as demanded by healthcare providers to aid and reduce nosocomial infections in the healthcare setting.

It may be that ice from ice makers is not to be used for human consumption within the healthcare setting, but is suitable for medical purposes, e.g. for use in ice packs to reduce swelling. In those instances the ice packs and ice makers should be clearly labelled identifying intended use. This ice should not be mixed with ice that has been made in the freezer section of a domestic fridge as the latter is clearly for human consumption only.

Best practice for the use of water coolers and ice makers

- The advice of the infection prevention and control team (IPCT) and hospital engineering/estates department should be sought prior to purchasing new water coolers/ice makers.
- Both the IPCT and the hospital engineering department/estates should keep an inventory of all ice makers and water coolers within the healthcare setting.
- A maintenance programme/contract should be set up with the hospital engineering department/estates and maintenance records kept.
- The siting of the machine should be in an area that is free from obstruction and where the air inlet and air outlet of the heat exchange unit allows for efficient cooling. The water reservoir and ice storage compartment should be well insulated.
- All new water coolers and ice makers should be plumbed into the mains water supply. Drainage from the unit requires a U-bend and a break to prevent reflux.
- All moving parts should be easily removable to promote cleaning. Cleaning should be done weekly. Any ice left over should be discarded. The unit should be cleaned with hot water and detergent using a disposable cloth followed by a thorough rinse using potable water and then with sodium

hypochlorite 100ppm. Allow to dry before returning to use. Records must be kept of the cleaning schedule.

- On a quarterly basis, and in accordance with the manufacturer's instructions, all removable parts of the machine should be taken apart for further cleaning, checking also for breakages, wear and tear. Record of this should be kept.

- Water coolers with drip trays must be kept clean, dry and cleaned daily with detergent and hot water. It should be the responsibility of the ward/ department manager to ensure this is done. A daily log sheet must be maintained.

- Ice handlers should not handle ice with their hands; an impermeable scoop should be used. The scoop to remove the ice should be smooth and impervious and kept in an impervious lidded container. Both items should be cleaned at the end of each shift, further cleaned if visibly dirty, and sterilised daily.

- Ice handlers should decontaminate their hands immediately prior to and after dispensing the ice. Unused ice should not be returned to the ice storage compartment. Unused ice at the end of the day should be disposed of.

- The door to the ice storage compartment should be kept closed except when dispensing the ice.

- Ice makers should not be accessible to the public and should be clearly marked for staff handling only.

- Water coolers may require further external decontamination if situated in a busy hospital corridor.

- Ice for consumption should not be transported between wards or departments.

- All extraneous equipment and items should be removed from on or around the ice maker/water cooler.

- Recycling of excess water into the reservoir or ice storage compartment is not recommended.

- Personal water bottles should not be topped up from water coolers; water should not be taken directly from the machine, i.e. as though it was a fountain, and only single use cups should be used.

- Adherence to the Food Safety Act 1990 and all current legislation must be maintained.

The following recommendations are suggested by Peterson (1982), Burnett et al (1994), Gallagher (1999) and current legislation.

Patients who have certain conditions or are undergoing particular treatments can become immunocompromised. Such a simple pleasure as having an iced drink or being able to suck on a soothing ice cube can become life threatening.

Wilson et al (1997) say that 'neutropenic patients are at particular risk if they are allowed to suck ice cubes which have sharp edges as they may lacerate the oral mucosa which has been compromised by therapeutic regimens'. Neutropenic patients are often encouraged to drink sterile water and such patients should not be given ice from an ice maker. Ice for these patients should be made by putting sterile water into single use ice makers in a conventional freezer (NHS Estates 2002).

Another method used by staff to help cool patients was to place a bowl of ice beneath an electric fan. However, this is no longer recommended as the potential for aerosolisation of water-borne pathogens is high (Burnett et al 1994).

Serious consideration must be given to the following when deciding to purchase a water cooler or ice maker:

- Is the appliance user-friendly?
- What is its intended purpose, e.g. is it for staff or patients?
- Confirm that routine maintenance is allotted to a specific person who will take on this role. How will the task will be continued in his/her absence?
- Develop a standard operating procedure to ensure all staff follow the correct maintenance and cleaning process and documentation.
- Agree with staff (including the IPCT and estates/engineering departments) and users the most appropriate place for it in the department.

Key points

- All staff and service users who access the water cooler/ice maker must observe good hand hygiene
- The purpose of the ice/water cooler must be clarified and adhered to, e.g. is it for medical use or staff/patient consumption?
- It is vital to keep a maintenance log of the appliance
- Ensure there is an updated cleaning schedule available
- Keep up to date with the policies and guidelines around the use of the appliance
- Ensure the ice maker has a smooth impermeable scoop and is kept in a lidded container

---

As a consequence of limited storage space and the need to reduce any potential water-borne infections the IPCT should advise departmental managers who wish to purchase water coolers/ice makers that they are plumbed directly into the mains water supply as opposed to the stand alone type. The latter should be phased out when they are judged unfit for use by environmental audits.

Some wards or departments within the healthcare setting are only open from Monday to Friday. Furthermore, some trusts only open certain wards temporarily to relieve winter pressures or to reduce waiting lists. If these areas have a water cooler or ice machine it should be the responsibility of the manager who opens or closes these areas to ensure the machines are emptied, drained and cleaned and covered ready for next use. Any water allowed to remain in the pipework could be subjected to a growth of biofilm. Gebo et al (2002) advise that:

Knowledge of the growth of these organisms in water supplies has been greatly enhanced by a better understanding of biofilms, which are a filmy layer at the interface of the solid pipe and liquid phase of the water and which are a common source of growth of both bacteria and mycobacteria.

If a ward or department is only open for a short period of time over the year it may be more prudent to remove the machines altogether, thereby reducing that potential source of water-borne infection.

Prevention of *Legionella*

Legionnaires' disease is caused by the bacterium *Legionella pneumophilia* which can be found in environmental water sources and water systems, particularly those in larger buildings such as hotels, office blocks and hospitals. For disease to occur the bacterium needs to be aerosolised such as from cooling towers, evaporative condensers, whirlpool spas and shower heads. Pneumonia can develop after the bacterium is inhaled and individuals over the age of 50 years, smokers, diabetics and those that are immunocompromised are at greater risk.

Legionella spp. embed into the sediment, sludge and biofilms of water tanks and pipes, which provide the ideal growth requirements. The organisms can readily grow at temperatures of between 20°C–45°C; the biofilms, sludge and scale protect the organism against adverse temperatures and biocides that would normally kill or inhibit them. It is estimated that 12–85% of hospital water systems are colonised with legionella.

Box 8.1. Risk assessment for exposure to legionnaires' disease and other illnesses

- Are conditions right for the bacteria to multiply, e.g. is the water temperature between 20°C and 45°C?
- Are there areas where stagnant water occurs (dead legs), e.g. pipes to a washing machine that is no longer used?
- Are there infrequently used outlets, e.g. showers, taps?
- Is there debris in the system, such as rust, sludge or scale (often a problem in old metal cisterns), that could provide food for growing *Legionella*?
- Are there thermostatic mixing valves that set a favourable outlet temperature for *Legionella* growth?
- Are any of your employees, residents, visitors, etc. vulnerable to infection, e.g. older people, those already ill?

Answering 'yes' to any of these questions suggests there is an increased risk of your patients/residents being exposed to legionella and falling ill.

The Approved Code of Practice and guidance for Legionnaires disease (Health and Safety Executive 2000) outlines the need to carry out risk assessments in all residential accommodation to comply with the legislation (Health and Safety Executive 2000). The risk assessment is outlined in *Box 8.1*.

Since the majority of healthcare settings and all hospitals will have one or more of the risks identified in *Box 8.1*, steps must be taken to prevent illness. The hospital's or healthcare organisation's estates department should have a policy to manage the risks to prevent *Legionella* affecting patients, staff and visitors (Department of Health 2009a).

Contamination of the water supply can occur due to poor design of pipework, inappropriate storage of water or during renovation and refurbishment (NHS Estates 2002). These problems can be overcome by regular cleaning of the water storage tanks; maintaining a consistently high temperature in the water supply; introducing a form of online disinfection, such as chlorine dioxide, if the temperature cannot be maintained; minimising dead legs; removing unused pipework and appliances; performed regular water system maintenance; and minimising water storage.

In an independent review of suppression of *Legionella* in hospitals and other healthcare establishments, the Department of Health (2009b) stated that raising the temperature of hot water effectively reduces the viable concentration of *Legionella* spp. but the organism persists in cooler water in taps, showers and dead legs. The review favours ionisation or chlorine dioxide over heat, with chlorine dioxide being more effective against biofilm. The review concludes that when considering efficacy, reliability and energy costs, copper/silver ionisation or chlorine dioxide technologies should be recommended but acknowledges the need for adequate monitoring to be in place.

Further guidance on control of *Legionella* in water systems can be found in the Health and Safety Executive's (2000) Approved Code of Practice and Guidance. Part 1 of this publication contains advice on healthcare workers' duties under the law and Part 2 contains guidance on the technical aspects of the assessment and control of *Legionella* risks.

Summary

In this chapter we have examined the principles of safe food and water handling in order to prevent infections due to contamination. We have looked at the components of best practice and discussed some of the main infections which have occurred due to poor hygiene. We have learned the importance of documentation, hand hygiene and maintenance in order to ensure safe care for patients. In the next chapter we will look at this further in relation to the medical devices used in the patient care.

Case study

There have been numerous high profile hospital outbreaks of infection resulting from both food-borne and water-borne sources. Probably the most notable food-borne outbreak was at Stanley Royd Hospital, Wakefield in 1984 when *Salmonella* spp. affected 355 patients and 102 staff and resulted in 19 deaths (Department of Health and Social Security 1986).

- Consider what actions you will take to prevent further spread of an outbreak.
- How will you support the patients affected by this?

References

Ayliffe GAJ, Babb JR, Taylor LJ (1999) *Hospital-acquired infection. Principles and prevention* (3rd edn, pp 118–19). Butterworth Heinemann, Oxford

Bangsborg JM, Uldum S, Jenson JS, Bruun BG (1995) Nosocomial legionellosis in three heart-lung transplant patients: Case reports and environmental observations. *European Journal of Clinical Microbiology and Infectious Diseases* **14**: 99–104

Burnett IA, Weeks GR, Harris DM (1994) A hospital study of ice-making machines: Their bacteriology, design, usage and upkeep. *Journal of Hospital Infection* **28**: 305–13

Cotton MF, Wasserman E, Pieper CH, Theron DG, van Tubbergh D, Campbell G, Fang FC, Barnes J (2000) Invasive disease due to extended spectrum beta-lactamase producing *Klebsiella pneumoniae* in a neonatal unit: The possible role of cockroaches. *Journal of Hospital Infection* **44**(1): 13–17

Department of Health (2009a) *Health and Social Care Act 2008.* Available from: www. opsi.gov.uk/acts/acts2008/pdf/ukpga_20080014_en.pdf

Department of Health (2009b) *Independent review of evidence regarding selection of techniques for the suppression of* Legionella *in water supplies of hospitals and other healthcare premises.* Available from: www.dh.gov.uk/prod_consum_dh/groups/ dh_digitalassets/documents/digitalasset/dh_102861.pdf [Accessed 10 April 2010]

Department of Health and Social Security (1986) *Report on the Committee of Enquiry into an outbreak of food poisoning at Stanley Royd Hospital.* Her Majesty's Stationary Office, London

Food Standards Agency (1990) *The Food Safety Act 1990 – A guide for food businesses.* Available from: http://www.food.gov.uk/multimedia/pdfs/fsactguide.pdf [Accessed 10 April 2010]

Food Standards Agency (2005) *Safer Food Better Business. FSA/0993/0905.* Food Standards Agency, London

Gallagher R (1999) Cold comfort. *Nursing Times* **95**(2): 55–6

Gebo KA, Srinivasan A, Perl TM, Ross T, Groth A, Merz WG (2002) Pseudo-outbreak of *Mycobacterium fortuitum* on a human immunodeficiency virus ward: Transient respiratory tract colonization from a contaminated ice machine. *Clinical Infectious Diseases* **35**: 32–8

Graman PS, Quinlan GA, Rank JA (1997) *Nosocomial Legionellosis* traced to a contaminated ice machine. *Infection Control and Hospital Epidemiology* **18**(9): 637–40

Hall J, Hodgson G, Kerr KG (2004) Provision of safe potable water for immunocompromised patients in hospital. *Journal of Hospital Infection* **58**: 155–8

Health Protection Agency (2010a) *Enteric routine data reports.* Available from: http://www.hpa.org.uk/hpr/infections/enteric.htm#gofiQ309 [Accessed 5 April 2010]

Health Protection Agency (2010b) *Legionnaires' disease: Epidemiological data.* Available from: http://www.hpa.org.uk/Topics/InfectiousDiseases/InfectionsAZ/LegionnairesDisease/EpidemiologicalData/ [Accessed 5 April 2010]

Health and Safety Executive (2000) *Legionnaires' disease. The control of Legionella bacteria in water systems. Approved Code of Practice and Guidance L8* (3rd edn). HSE Books, London

Laussucq S, Baltch AL, Smith RP et al (1988) Nosocomial *Mycobacterium fortuitum* colonization from a contaminated ice machine. *American Reviews of Respiratory Disease* **138**: 891–4

National Patient Safety Agency (2007) *Clean Safe Care posters.* NPSA, London

NHS Estates (2002) *Infection control in the built environment: Design and planning HFN 30* (2nd edn). The Stationery Office, Norwich

Peterson NJ (1982) Don't culture ice machines. *Hospital Infection Control* 9: 8–9

Pia H, Chen W, Peng C (2004) Cockroaches as potential vectors of nosocomial infection. *Infection Control and Hospital Epidemiology* **25**: 979–84

Pratt RJ, Pellowe CM, Wilson JA, Loveday HP, Harper PJ, Jones SRLJ, McDougall C, Wilcox MH (2007) Epic2: National evidence-based guidelines for preventing healthcare-associated infections in NHS hospitals in England. *Journal of Hospital Infection* **65**(Suppl 1): S1–S64

Schuetz AN, Hughes RL, Howard RM et al (2009) Pseudo-outbreak of *Legionella pneumophila* Serogroup 8 infection associated with a contaminated ice machine in a bronchoscopy suite. *Infection Control and Hospital Epidemiology* **30**(5): 461–6

Stout JE, Lin YE, Goetz AM, Muder RR (1998) Controlling *Legionella* in hospital water systems: Experience with the superheat-and-flush method and copper-silver ionization. *Infection Control and Hospital Epidemiology* **19**: 911–14

Stout JE, Yu VL, Muraca P (1985) Isolation of *Legionella pneumophila* from the cold water of hospital ice machines: Implications for origin and transmission of the organism. *Infection Control* **6**(4): 141–6

Wall PG, Ryan MJ, Ward LR, Rowe B (1996) Outbreaks of salmonellosis in hospitals in England and Wales 1992–1994. *Journal of Hospital Infection* **33**: 181–90

WHO (2006) *Guidelines on hand hygiene in health care. First Global Patient Safety*

Challenge. Clean Care is Safer Care. WHO, Geneva

Wilson IG, Hogg GM, Barr JG (1997) Microbiological quality of ice in hospital and community. *Journal of Hospital Infection* **36**: 171–80

Suggested further reading

Bencini MA, Yzerman PF, Koornstra RHT et al (2005) A case of Legionnaires' disease caused by aspiration of ice water. *Archives of Environmental and Occupational Health* **60**(6): 302–6

Ravn P, Lundgren J D, Kjaeldgaard P et al (1991) Nosocomial outbreak of cryptosporidiosis in AIDS patients. *British Medical Journal* **302**: 277–80

Wilson J (2006) *Infection control in clinical practice* (3rd edn, pp 84–5). Bailliere-Tindall, Edinburgh

Section 3

Management and treatment

CHAPTER 9

Management of invasive devices

Annette Jeanes

Purpose

This chapter looks at some of the invasive devices used within healthcare and how to reduce the risks of infections through their safe management.

Learning outcomes

By the end of the chapter, you will have learned

- Some of the key medical devices uses within healthcare.
- The infection risks associated with the devices.
- The role of asepsis and decontamination in caring for the devices and the client.
- The safe management of devices.

Introduction

The use of invasive devices in the delivery of healthcare is common, particularly in acute care. Devices that breach the protective barriers and defences of the body, such as the skin, are invasive and are a particular risk of infection. They offer an opportunity for microorganisms to be introduced at insertion, during the time they are in place, and at and after removal. Invasive devices increase the risk of infection in patients and their use should be avoided if possible. In some instances non-invasive devices are available and should be used in preference.

Invasive devices

An invasive device breaches the normal barriers of the body, such as the skin and sphincters. Examples of invasive devices include:

- Central venous catheters.
- Peripheral arterial lines.

Box 9.1. Functions of invasive devices

Invasive devices have numerous functions including:
* Administration of drugs, food or fluids
* Monitoring and measuring, e.g. blood gases and blood pressure
* Support or stabilisation
* Drainage

---

* Peripheral intravenous devices.
* Epidural and spinal infusion devices.
* Urinary catheters.
* Wound and chest drains.
* External ventricular drains.
* Tracheostomy tubes.
* Gastrostomy tubes.
* Peritoneal dialysis catheters.

The functions of different devices are shown in *Box 9.1*.

Infection risks of invasive devices

Generally, hospitalised patients are exposed to a greater risk of infection than patients in the community and invasive devices are a factor in this increased risk. However, invasive devices are increasingly being used in community settings. Common factors that increase the risk of infection are shown in *Box 9.2*.

The risk of infection is usually increased with the length of time the device is in place (Elliott 1988). This is often referred to as the 'dwell time'. There are some exceptions where devices, such as midline catheters, are designed for long-term use. Various underlying factors affect the vulnerability of patients to infection, including device-related infection; these include age, immune status and underlying condition. The composition, design and type of device are other influencing factors. Frequent manipulation, disconnection, blockage and backflow also contribute to an increased risk of infection.

The initial insertion of a device may cause trauma or damage that can allow microorganisms to enter the body. Male catheterisation, for example, can be particularly traumatic. It is important to ensure that all healthcare

---

Box 9.2. Factors that increase the risk of infection

The following factors increase the risk of infection:
- The patient's immune status
- The patient's underlying condition
- Increased manipulation of the medical device
- Prolonged use of the device

---

workers inserting invasive devises are trained and competent in the procedure to reduce the risks of insertion trauma. Patients also have a role to play in reducing the risk of infection and should be made aware of the insertion process, what they may feel during insertion, and what they can do to minimise risks of infection.

The subsequent care and removal of the device are important as microorganisms may be introduced during manipulation and sampling. The presence of a device in the body prompts a physiological response including the creation of a biofilm on the surface of the device (Kurladze 2007). The device may become a reservoir of microorganisms and a source of infection.

Prevention of infection

The prevention of infection in invasive devices is summarised in *Box 9.3* and begins by avoiding the use of invasive devices unless it is absolutely necessary.

Box 9.3. Prevention of infection in invasive devices

- Avoid use of invasive device if possible
- Remove the device as soon as possible
- Educate and train inserters
- Use aseptic technique
- Perform hand hygiene before and after handling device
- Use sterile equipment
- Clean the insertion site
- Monitor for signs of inflammation or infection
- Document insertion and removal

If an invasive device is required, it should be removed as soon as it is no longer needed, as the presence of the device increases the risk of acquiring and developing an infection.

Staff inserting invasive devices should be educated, skilled and competent in insertion. Training and practice should begin with manikins or models rather than patients, as initial insertions may be clumsy and can cause pain and trauma.

An aseptic technique should be used during insertion for most procedures. Sterile barrier precautions are required for particularly invasive procedures such as insertion of central venous catheters. The handling of devices, and sampling and manipulating the equipment associated with the device also require care and attention to asepsis and hand hygiene.

Asepsis

Some situations and procedures increase the potential for the introduction of microorganisms to the patient, including the insertion of invasive devices. Asepsis aims to minimise the presence of pathogenic microorganisms in the clinical setting and is the principle of preventing the introduction of infection during a procedure or intervention. Aseptic technique utilises the principles of asepsis to protect the patient from the introduction of infection and can be used in a variety of settings. The checklist in *Box 9.4* provides an overview of the key points to include when undertaking an aseptic technique.

Asepsis is used in a range of activities. The highest levels of asepsis are used in operating theatres. A series of measures need to be taken including frequent air exchange and air filtration; use of sterile drapes, equipment, gloves and surfaces; surgical scrubbing; use of disinfectants; and separation of sterile and non-sterile fields. Healthcare staff normally wear clean low lint theatre clothing; hair is covered and further personal protective equipment, sometimes including face masks, is recommended. This all contributes to a reduction in microorganisms near the patient.

In other clinical areas or situations, similar levels of asepsis may not be achievable or appropriate. A sterile barrier technique may be used, which includes performing a surgical scrub, gowning, draping, wearing gloves, and using sterile equipment and an aseptic technique. This may be appropriate in, for example, the insertion of a central venous catheter. Procedures such as urinary catheterisation do not require this level of asepsis and it is sufficient to use scrupulous hand hygiene, sterile equipment, sterile gloves and a non-touch technique.

Box 9.4. Checklist for aseptic technique

☐ Use sterile equipment, fluids and drugs
☐ Ensure the area where the procedure is to take place is as clean as possible
☐ Ensure minimal disruption occurs during the procedure which would lead to air turbulence and dust distribution
☐ Clean hands thoroughly before and during the procedure if contamination occurs. In particular invasive procedures a surgical scrub is required
☐ Prepare the setting, including decontamination of the dressing trolley or surface with detergent and water, and then dry. Next disinfect the surface with a 70% alcohol wipe
☐ Assemble everything required before starting, to reduce the need to leave the patient and sterile field during the procedure
☐ Minimise contamination of the site by use of sterile gloves or forceps and/or by not touching sterile parts of the equipment (non-touch technique)
☐ Create a sterile field to work on. This is normally a sterile towel which is laid out without contaminating the centre and only touching the edges
☐ Avoid contaminating the sterile field created to undertake the procedure
☐ Discard single use equipment and products after use and do not reuse
☐ Avoid contamination of the sterile field. Once an item is contaminated, discard away from the sterile field. This is often referred to as going from clean to dirty and is used throughout the process
☐ Wear appropriate personal protective equipment. A plastic disposable apron should be worn over clothing or uniform to form a barrier, to avoid contamination of the sterile field and to prevent contamination of clothing. Disposable gloves should be worn when contact with body substances is anticipated

---

Hand hygiene

Hands must be cleaned before and after each patient contact, and after any task that may have resulted in the hands becoming contaminated. This is reflected in the World Health Organization 'Five moments of hand hygiene' (see *Figure 4.2, Chapter 4*) (WHO 2009). Handling any device requires scrupulous attention to hand hygiene and may also require the use of sterile gloves. Disposable gloves should always be worn when contact with body substances is anticipated. The use of gloves does not preclude hand hygiene. Hands should be cleaned prior to and after the use of gloves. Disposable gloves are single use and should not be decontaminated with alcohol or any other substance.

It is preferable to wash hands with soap and water at a clinical hand washing sink before commencing a procedure that requires an aseptic technique. If hands are not contaminated, subsequent hand hygiene during the procedure with alcohol or other decontaminants is sufficient (WHO 2009).

Sterile equipment

The use of sterile equipment, including fluids and drugs, reduces the potential for contamination. Invasive devices are normally sterile and will have been through a validated decontamination process. It is important to ensure the equipment is stored adequately to reduce any damage, particularly penetration by water and alteration caused by heat or light. Prior to use the integrity of packaging and the 'use by' date should be checked.

Items are frequently single use and should be discarded after one use. This includes lotions, anaesthetic gels, dressings and gloves. Some equipment is reusable and can be decontaminated before reuse, e.g. laryngeal masks. Local decontamination should not take place in healthcare facilities unless the process has been formally validated as safe and effective. The decontamination process must meet national regulatory requirements and be documented.

Insertion site preparation and care

Preparation is to some extent specific to the site and device used but the general principals are:

- The site should be as clean as possible.
- The device should be secure and stable following insertion.
- There should be minimal disruption and manipulation of the site.
- Where the skin is breached a sterile dressing is normally required.

Observation of the insertion site and examination of the securing system and/or dressing used should be undertaken regularly. This is to detect any inflammation, exudate and other signs that may indicate infection or malfunction. Dressings or securing systems vary in how frequently they require changing but generally disruption or disturbance should be avoided.

Composition and design of devices

The composition and design of a device vary with its type and function. In general, the design and composition of devices attempts to offer as few opportunities for the introduction and colonisation of microorganisms as possible. Some devices are impregnated with an antimicrobial substance or antibiotic which reduces the risk of infection. This additional technology particularly assists in the reduction of biofilm which may support bacterial growth while the device is in use. Other devices are engineered to prevent occlusion, reduce back flow and minimise irritation and discomfort.

The need for regular replacement varies with devices and may be affected by the material used, which includes silicone, Teflon, latex and polyurethane. Most devices have agreed standards that detail how long they can remain in place and how often they need to be replaced.

Many devices have secondary components such as collection bags or tubing. These should be compatible with the device and connected securely.

Documentation

Documentation should record the reason for, and date and time of insertion, details of the device and subsequent management, including removal. It is also helpful to record who undertook the procedure and if an aseptic or total barrier technique was used. Sometimes devices are inserted in an emergency and it is not possible to adopt all the recommended preventative measures; in this case, it is helpful to identify these devices since early removal and replacement may be required. Details of what should be documented are shown in *Box 9.5*.

Box 9.5. Documentation

Accurate documentation is important when caring for a patient with a medical device. Always ensure the following is documented:
- The date of insertion
- Who inserted the medical device
- Whether it was inserted in an emergency situation
- Any signs of infections
- When it was removed

Observation for signs of infection, dislodgement, malfunction, pain and any other relevant issues should be recorded and reported as necessary. Removal of the device should also be recorded. Some devices have a potential to degrade and it is important to inspect removed devices and confirm they have been removed in their entirety. Retained devices or parts of devices may lead to infection or other complications (Tindall et al 2002, Espiritu and Stolar 2007).

Management of an indwelling device

The management of an indwelling device should be optimised to ensure the risks of introduction of microorganisms to the patient are minimised. This varies with the type and function of the device. The preparation of a clean site for insertion and subsequent care has already been mentioned. Devices that are fundamentally hollow tubes usually require maintenance to ensure patency and to prevent blockage. Each time the device is accessed there is an opportunity to introduce microorganisms. It is therefore important that asepsis and sterile equipment are used at all times and that the integrity of the device or system is not breached.

The use of flushes and washouts have the potential for the introduction of contaminants with the flushing of debris from the device into the patient's system (Rao and Elliot 1988, Held et al 2006). This type of procedure should be undertaken with care and where possible a closed system should be utilised. A similar issue may arise with sampling and flushing.

Secondary equipment such as bungs, additional tubing and bags also require careful management and are device specific. The same scrupulous hand hygiene measures and asepsis should be applied, and contamination avoided by careful decontamination.

Management using evidence-based guidance

There is a considerable body of evidence associated with preventing device-related infection. In England, the Saving Lives programme was launched in 2005 and has a number of evidence-based bundles which, if applied, will reduce the risk of infection (Department of Health 2007). Similar programmes were also developed in Wales and Scotland.

Many invasive devices have specific evidence-based guidance but this chapter now focuses on intravenous and urinary catheter devices as they are the most commonly used.

Box 9.6. Examples of intravenous access devices

- Central venous catheters (CVC)
- Peripheral venous catheters
- Midline catheters
- Peripherally inserted central catheters (PICC)
- Implanted intravascular devices

Intravenous access devices

Intravenous devices are hollow tubes that allow access to the vascular system. Examples are shown in *Box 9.6*.

Intravenous and arterial devices share many features but vary in their usage; venous devices are generally used to give infusions while arterial devices are usually used for monitoring and blood testing. The frequent manipulation of arterial devices, particularly with pressure monitoring systems, may increase the risk of infection. The following explanation concentrates on intravenous devices but devices placed in arteries require similar management.

Types of infection

Intravenous catheters are associated with a significant risk of bacteraemia, particularly central lines. Bacteraemia is the presence of infection in the bloodstream and infections related to intravenous catheters are sometimes referred to as catheter-related bloodstream infections (CRBSIs). These infections increase both the average length of hospital stay and the risk of death (Pittet et al 1994). Diagnosis is usually by blood culture and the microorganisms responsible are often from skin or other patient flora but may be introduced by the healthcare worker. Methicillin-resistant *Staphylococcus aureus* (MRSA) is a particular risk.

Phlebitis is a local inflammation of the vein and tissue at the insertion site. Early signs are redness and soreness but phlebitis may develop with symptoms of swelling and pus. A more generalised infection, such as bacteraemia, may occur when microorganisms from the skin and insertion site enter the bloodstream by migrating along the device.

163

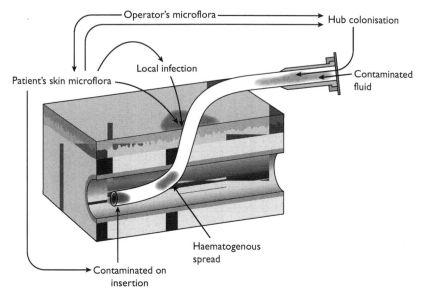

Figure 9.1. Routes of infection in intravenous catheters.

Routes of infection

The routes of infection are illustrated in *Figure 9.1*. The usual points of entry of microorganisms are at insertion and then subsequently by travelling through or along the outside of the intravenous catheter. The surface of the skin is usually colonised with microorganisms and these may be introduced through the skin or into the blood vessel during insertion. Microorganisms may originate from the inserter or subsequent healthcare workers' hands. Bacteria may also travel along the outside of the intravenous catheter from the insertion site. Handling of the line and the introduction of drugs or fluids may also introduce microorganisms, either by contaminated infusate or via a contaminated hub or device, such as a three-way tap. Haematogenous spread occurs when microorganisms that are already present in the blood become attached and multiply on the line, particularly the tip. These may then be released back into the bloodstream to cause infection (Donlan 2001).

Prevention of infection

In facilities where intravenous devices are used, guidelines for insertion and management should be available. The focus of prevention is to reduce the opportunities to introduce pathogens. The key aspects of prevention are outlined in *Box 9.7.*

Box 9.7. Key steps to prevent infection in patients with an intravenous access device

- Avoid insertion of a device unless absolutely necessary, and remove as soon as possible
- Ensure inserter is suitably trained and competent
- Ensure skin antisepsis at insertion
- Perform insertion using asepsis
- Ensure good hand hygiene and aseptic technique when handling device and connections
- Inform the patient of the process
- Use sterile equipment and supplies
- Use sterile infusate and intravenous injections
- Avoid contamination of hubs and connections
- Handle device as little as possible
- Maintain patency by flushing when not in use
- Secure the device to avoid dislodging it
- Document and monitor device

Training and competence of inserter

All staff who insert intravenous devices should be trained in the procedure and understand the associated risks. Staff who regularly and competently insert intravenous devices have been found to have a lower risk of infection (Boulamiery-Verry et al 2004). Increasingly, insertion teams and specialists undertake this role, with significant benefits (Soiffe et al 1998, Palefski and Stoddard 2001, Jackson 2007).

Skin antisepsis

To reduce the risk of colonisation or the introduction of microorganisms at the insertion site careful cleaning of the skin is necessary (Maki et al 1991).

The use of 2% chlorhexidine in 70% isopropyl alcohol is recommended (Pratt et al 2007) except in neonates when a 0.5% aqueous solution of 5% chlorhexidine is widely used. In patients with sensitivity to chlorhexidine, povidone-iodine may be used. The skin should be cleaned with the solution prior to insertion and allowed to dry for approximately 30 seconds. No further unsterile palpations of the prepared site should then take place during insertion.

Environment

A well-lit and well-ventilated environment is preferable. During insertion, there should be enough room to gain access to the patient allowing unrestricted movement without the risk of knocks. Some procedures require more than one person and there should be room to create and maintain a sterile field.

Insertion of some lines, such as central venous catheters, implantable devices and pulmonary arterial catheters, require additional equipment such as ultrasound and x-ray. It may be preferable to undertake these insertions in theatre or other specialist environment, particularly as they require a high level of sterility and asepsis.

Type of device

Devices are normally single use and delivered sterile in packs. The device used should be as small as possible in diameter and length to reduce trauma but take into account the purpose for which it is to be used and the size of the vessel to be cannulated. Typically, rapid infusions of blood will require large-bore devices.

Antimicrobial impregnated devices have been shown to reduce infection rates, particularly in high risk patients (Maki et al 1997).

Cannulae are hollow bore needles which may hold large amounts of blood and are a significant risk in the transmission of blood-borne virus. Safety engineered devices which reduce the risk of needlestick injury are available.

Tunnelled devices are recommended for patients who require long-term intravenous access since the risk of infection is reduced, they may be more comfortable and patients may be able to manage them at home.

A single lumen is preferable to multiple lumens since the latter increase the risk of infection, in part because each extra lumen increases the potential for contamination (Dezfulian et al 2003). However, in some patients, multiple lumen access is preferable as it makes care delivery more efficient.

Device replacement

The routine replacement of devices should be avoided. The continued requirement for a device should be assessed at least daily and if it is no longer required it should be removed (Department of Health 2007).

Peripheral cannulas should be removed as soon as possible. Many institutions have policies that recommend the replacement of these devices in a new site after 72 to 96 hours or earlier if clinically indicated. While it is rational to remove the device if it is malfunctioning, painful or inflamed, there is little evidence that routine replacement reduces infection (Webster et al 2010). In some instances where venous access is difficult and the device is functioning with no signs of complications or pain it may stay in place longer.

The risk of infection in central venous catheters increases with each day of catheterisation (Elliott 1988). Catheters should therefore be removed as soon as possible and not routinely replaced unless they are required. The manufacturer's guidance on replacement should be followed and some devices, such as tunnelled devices, are designed for long-term use.

Set and tubing replacement

Administration sets used for blood and blood products should be changed immediately following the transfusion. Some drug infusions also require the immediate changing of sets following administration. Sets used for total parenteral nutrition, which contains lipids, should be changed after 24 hours. Other sets used for the administration of intravenous fluids should be used for a maximum of 72 to 96 hours and then discarded (Gilles et al 2005). Any set that is temporarily disconnected should be capped with a sterile device to prevent contamination.

Access to the intravenous line

Aseptic technique should be used for any access to or handling of the line. The use of 2% chlorhexidine in 70% isopropyl alcohol is recommended for cleaning catheter ports or hubs prior to accessing the line for administering fluids or injections (Pratt et al 2007). Access should be limited as frequent use increases the risk of contamination. Catheter injection ports should be covered by caps or valved connectors. Hubs, ports, connectors and three-way taps may become contaminated (Seymou et al 2000). Needle-free connectors and extension devices reduce the risk of contamination although they have been implicated in increased line-related infections with fluids such as parenteral nutrition (Danzig et al 1995).

Infusate and additives

Infusions and substances added may become contaminated or colonised but this is rare (Rickard et al 2009). Intravenous fluids are usually produced under aseptic conditions. Contamination usually takes place during use and to combat this filters may be used. The use of multiple-use vials has been implicated in the transmission of infection and should be avoided (Mattner and Gastmeier 2004). Scrupulous hand hygiene is essential when handling intravenous lines and infusion sets.

Flushing

The prevention of blockage, particularly in devices that are not in continuous use, is normally with a flush of sterile saline, water or heparin. There is evidence that instilling and leaving a 'lock' of heparin, alcohol or antibiotics may reduce the risk of bacteraemia but this is currently not routinely used (Raad et al 2008). It is currently recommended that a positive pressure with a pulsating flush is used since this achieves optimal results (Royal College of Nursing 2010).

Selection of site of insertion

Peripheral cannulas should be inserted in the non-dominant limb avoiding joints as this allows the patient to move and avoids dislodgement. It is recommended in the UK that central venous catheters are inserted in the sub-clavian or internal jugular vein (Hamilton and Foxcroft 2007) although for some patients, e.g. those undergoing neurosurgery, a femoral site is often preferred. Although the risk of infection is higher in femoral catheters, specific requirements, such as surgery involving the upper torso, may determine where lines are sited.

Dressing

An adherent sterile, semi-permeable dressing, preferably with a clear central panel to observe the site, is recommended. This provides protection, stability and visibility. It should be kept dry and intact. There is evidence that the application of antiseptic impregnated dressings to the site and the use of fixation devices to ensure the device is stable, reduce the risk of infection (Ho and Litton 2006, Schears 2006). A label giving details of the date and time of insertion should be used.

Documentation

The date of and rationale for insertion should be recorded in the patient's notes to assist in communication about the purpose of the line and when it should be removed.

The method of insertion and details of the device should also be recorded, including site of insertion, type of device and gauge. The requirement for continued use of an intravenous device should be checked regularly and it should be removed as soon as possible. This should be recorded. Signs of infection should also be recorded and reported.

Monitoring of the insertion site and device

The site should be observed at least daily for signs of infection or dysfunction. Simple and consistent documentation using a scoring system such as the Visual Infusion Phlebitis Score (VIPS) system, which is a tool to monitor infusion entry sites and to detect signs of infection (Jackson 1998), should be used. This ensures a standard approach is applied to assessment and recording of findings. If there is evidence of infection the line should be removed as soon as possible.

Key points to consider when caring for intravenous lines

* Skin asepsis
* Environment cleanliness
* Replacement of device
* Replacement of set and tubing
* Access to intravenous line
* Infusate – adding and flushing
* Intravenous site dressing

Urinary catheters

Urinary catheters are drainage tubes that are inserted into the bladder, normally through the urethra although supra-pubic catheters may be inserted directly into the bladder. Intermittent catheters may be used to drain urine but most devices are indwelling and are designed to be left in place. Indwelling urinary catheters are attached to drainage bags which collect the urine.

Types of device

Urinary catheters include:

* Standard indwelling urinary catheter (Foley) with integral balloon.
* Short-term catheter with no balloon.

169

- Irrigation catheter for post-operative irrigation.
- Supra-pubic catheter.

Catheters may be made of a number of materials including latex, silicone and Teflon. Most catheters in hospitals are removed within 14 days (Brosnanhan et al 2004) and therefore the catheters most frequently selected are designed for short-term use (Robinson 2006). Long-term catheters remain in place for longer than 28 days and up to 12 weeks (Ward et al 1997). Silastic and polyvinylpyrolidone (PVP) catheters are recommended for long-term use (Nacey et al 1985, Berkov and Das 1998).

The formation of a biofilm is an important factor in the development of catheter-associated urinary tract infections (CAUTIs). To combat this some catheters contain or are coated in a variety of substances including antibiotics, antimicrobials or hydrogel and there is evidence that these contribute to reducing infection (Srinivasan et al 2006, Johnson et al 2006) .

There are a range of diameters and lengths. The diameter of catheters is measured using the Charriere (Ch) or French gauge scale which ranges from 3 to 34 Ch.

Shorter devices are used for females and smaller diameters are used in preference as they cause less urethral trauma, bladder spasm and pain (Nazarko 2009). The urinary catheter selected should be based on an individual patient assessment and if debris such as blood clots is anticipated, as this will require a higher gauge to prevent blockage.

Infection associated with urinary catheters

Catheter-associated urinary tract infections (CAUTIs) are one of the most common nosocomial infections (Health Protection Agency 2008) with the risk increasing with the length of time the catheter is in place (Maki and Tambyah 2001).

CAUTIs are frequently asymptomatic (Tambyah and Maki 2000) but symptoms may include a fever or chills, abdominal pain or tenderness, bloody or foul smelling urine, confusion, and obstruction or leakage of the catheter. It may cause pyelonephritis and can lead to bacteraemia. Localised urethral irritation and infection are also possible.

Diagnosis of a CAUTI is usually by urine sample which is examined in the microbiology department. The microorganisms responsible are frequently perineal flora. Gram-negative antibiotic resistant microorganisms are a particular risk. Treatment may include catheter removal and antibiotics.

Risks

The risk of developing an infection is increased with the length of time the catheter is in place. The relative risk of developing a urinary tract infection increases with each day of catheterisation and it is estimated that by 30 days infection is almost inevitable (Maki and Tambyah 2001). There is a higher risk of CAUTI in females and those with underlying conditions such as diabetes, renal insufficiency and malnutrition.

Figure 9.2 shows the route of infection in catheterised patients.

Routes of infection

The source and route of infection is generally from the patient's own flora or from contact with healthcare workers at insertion or during subsequent care. The meatus is normally colonised with microorganisms. There are two main routes, extra-luminal and intra-luminal, see *Figure 9.2*.

Extra-luminal contamination occurs during insertion or from the migration of microorganisms along the external surface of the catheter. Traumatic insertion may increase the risk of infection. It has been found that frequent meatal cleansing and manipulation of the catheter at the entry site may increase the risk of infection as it allows microorganisms to migrate along the outside of the tube (Burke et al 1981).

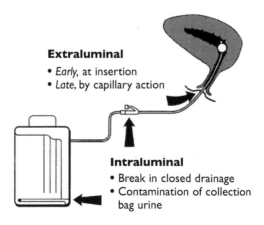

Extraluminal
- *Early*, at insertion
- *Late*, by capillary action

Intraluminal
- Break in closed drainage
- Contamination of collection bag urine

Figure 9.2. Route of infection in catheterised patients. Reproduced from Maki and Tambyah (2001) with permission.

Intra-luminal contamination is via the internal surface of the tubing and can result from contamination of the tubing, connections or bag. A biofilm rapidly develops on the surface of catheters (Saint and Chenoweth 2003) and this supports microorganisms which may be a source of infection, particularly during manipulation or reflux. This may occur during patient movement and whilst urine bags are emptied and their contents measured.

Prevention of infection

In facilities where urinary catheters are used, guidelines for insertion and management should be available. The focus of prevention is reducing the opportunities to introduce microorganisms. The key aspects of prevention are outlined in *Box 9.8.*

Alternatives, such as intermittent catheterisation and external urine collection devices, should be considered. If the insertion of a urinary catheter is essential, remove it as soon as it is no longer needed.

Box 9.8. Key points to prevent urinary infections

- Avoid urinary catheterisation if possible
- If it is essential remove the catheter as soon as it is no longer needed
- Consider alternatives, such as intermittent catheterisation and incontinence devices
- Use aseptic technique for insertion and subsequent care
- Catheters should be inserted by staff who are competent
- Use sterile equipment, gloves and drapes for insertion
- Clean the urethral meatus with sterile antiseptic or saline
- Use a single-use sterile local anaesthetic and lubricant for insertion
- Connect the catheter to a sterile closed drainage system
- Maintain the closed drainage system at all times
- Ensure downward drainage and prevent reflux
- Perform hand hygiene before and after handling the device
- Monitor for signs of inflammation or infection
- Document insertion and removal

Asepsis

The use of aseptic technique for insertion and subsequent care to prevent contamination of the device is well established. Sterile equipment, gloves and drapes for insertion should be used.

Training and competence of staff

Although intermittent catheterisation can be taught to patients, the insertion of an indwelling catheter is usually undertaken by a trained healthcare worker. Organisations that undertake this procedure should have protocols and guidelines on urinary catheter insertion. Many use recognised expert guidance such as the *Royal Marsden manual of clinical nursing procedures* (Dougherty and Lister 2008).

Environment

As with insertion of an intravenous access device, a well-lit and well-ventilated environment is preferable. During insertion, there should be enough room to gain access to the patient allowing unrestricted movement without the risk of knocks. More than one person may be required and there should be room to create and maintain a sterile field.

Insertion

The procedure should be explained to the patient to facilitate cooperation. Sterile equipment should be used with an aseptic technique. Hands should be cleaned scrupulously and sterile gloves worn for the insertion.

Clean the urethral meatus with sterile antiseptic or saline. Use a single use sterile local anaesthetic and lubricant for insertion in both males and females (Woodward 2005). Once the catheter is in place and secure, connect it to a sterile closed drainage system.

Product selection

Various technologies are available to help prevent infection although many are unproven, including anti-reflux valves (Maki and Tambyah 2001). Some, including antimicrobial and silver-impregnated catheters, do reduce the risk of infection (Schumm and Lam 2008) but may be more expensive than standard catheters. It is not clear currently if impregnated catheters are of value in long-term catheterisation.

Drainage system

A closed drainage system should be maintained at all times to prevent the introduction of microorganisms (Kunin and McCormack 1966). Disconnection for sampling and bag changes should be avoided if possible.

Ensure downward drainage and prevent reflux by positioning tubing and the urine collection bag below the level of the bladder at all times. Handling of the catheter and drainage bag should be minimised.

Documentation

The date and rationale for insertion should be recorded in notes to assist in communication about the purpose of the catheter and when it should be removed (Nazarko 2008). The method of insertion and details of the device should also be recorded, including the type of catheter and gauge. The requirement for a catheter should be checked regularly and it should be removed as soon as possible. This must be recorded as should the removal of the catheter. All catheter care should be documented. Signs of infection which may include pain and cloudy urine should also be recorded and reported.

Monitoring and surveillance

Monitoring and surveillance may vary in organisations but the monitoring of CAUTI is an indicator of standards of care. It is particularly useful to monitor trends in infection and microorganisms and to highlight catheters which are not required.

The prevalence of antibiotic-resistant microorganisms is increasing and is a particular problem in CAUTI. Advice from the infection control team may be required in the management of patients with antibiotic-resistant microorganisms.

Securement of urinary catheters

Various devices are available to secure the urinary catheter and tubing. The rationale is that this will prevent movement of the catheter and the potential to introduce microorganisms via the external lumen of the bladder. Although this is currently widely practised there is no clear evidence that it is effective. Securement devices may be a source of contamination if they are not maintained properly.

Supra-pubic catheter dressing

Supra-pubic catheters should be cleaned and a dry dressing applied daily until the site is healed and stable. The site should be monitored for signs of redness and inflammation.

Bladder washouts

Flushing of the bladder or washouts should be avoided if possible as they may introduce microorganisms and may damage the bladder (Rao and Elliot 1988). However, in some urological procedures, including surgery, this is routinely required to prevent blockage.

Box 9.10. Checklist for ongoing urinary catheter care

☐ Scrupulous hand hygiene whilst handling the urinary catheter and tubing is essential. It is particularly important to decontaminate hands before and after each patient contact. Wash or decontaminate hands and use disposable examination gloves if contact with body fluids is anticipated, e.g. emptying bags

☐ Maintain the catheter and attachments to minimise contamination. This should be detailed in local policies

☐ Clean the catheter insertion site regularly as part of the standard patient hygiene process

☐ If sampling is required this should be done aseptically via the catheter port

☐ Empty the drainage bag frequently to ensure the bladder can empty freely and to avoid backflow or reflux

☐ The drainage bag should always be positioned above the floor but below bladder level to prevent reflux or contamination

☐ Use a sterile jug or single use container for emptying the bag and do not use it for other patients

☐ Monitor the patient for signs of infection and remove the catheter as soon as possible if signs are present

☐ Document the care given and observations made

Catheter and bag replacement

Catheter bags should be changed according to manufacturers' recommendations. It is also important to change urinary catheters when clinically required and according to manufacturers' recommendations.

Summary

In this chapter we have looked at some of the key medical devices used within healthcare, focusing specifically on invasive intravenous access devices and urinary catheters. We examined aspects of care necessary to prevent infections and the importance of aseptic technique and documentation. In the next chapter we will build on this further by looking at other aspects of care that may be required by a patient with an infection.

References

Berkov S, Das S (1998) Urinary tract infection and intermittent catheterization. *Infections in Urology* **11**: 165–8

Boulamiery-Verry A, Mercia C, Duffand F, et al (2004) Totally implantable intravascular complications: Effectiveness of insertion by a trained team. *Journal of Hospital Infection* **56**(3): 248–9

Burke JP, Garibaldi RA ,Britt MR, et al (1981) Prevention of catheter-assocaied urinary tract infections: Efficacy of daily meatal care regimes. *American Journal of Medicine* **70**: 655–8

Brosnanhan J, Jull A, Tracy C (2004) Types of urethral catheters for management of short-term voiding problems in hospitalised adults. *Cochrane Database Systematic Review* CD004013

Danzig LE, Short L, Collins K, et al (1995) Bloodstream infections associated with a needleless intravenous infusion system and total partentral nutrition. *Journal of the American Medical Association* **273**: 1862–4

Department of Health (2007) *Saving Lives: Reducing infection, delivering clean and safe care*. Department of Health, London

Dezfulian, C, Lavelle, J, Nallamothu B, Kaufman S, Saint S (2003) Rates of infection for single-lumen versus multi-lumen central venous catheters: A meta-analysis. *Critical Care Medicine* **31**(9): 2385–90

Dougherty L, Lister S (eds) (2008) *The Royal Marsden manual of clinical nursing proce-*

dures. Wiley Blackwell, Chichester

Donlan RM (2001) Biofilms and device-associated infections. *Emerging Infectious Diseases Journal* 7(2): 277–81

Elliott TSJ (1988) Intravascular device infections. *Journal of Medical Microbiology* 27: 161–7

Espiritu JD, Stolar CG (2007) Pulmonary hypertension due to a retained totally implantable venous access device fragment. *Chest* 131(5): 1574–6

Gillies D, O'Riordan L, Wallen M, Morrison A, Rankin K, Nagy S (2005) Optimal timing for intravenous administration set replacement. *Cochrane Database Systematic Reviews* 19(4): CD003588

Hamilton HC, Foxcroft DR (2007) Central venous access sites for the prevention of venous thrombosis, syenosis and infection in patients requiring long-term intravenous therapy. *Cochrane Database Systematic Reviews* 3: CD004084

Health Protection Agency (2008) *Surveillance of healthcare associated infections report.* Health Protection Agency, London

Held MR, Begier EM, Beardsley DS, Browne FA, Martinello RA, et al (2006) Life-threatening sepsis caused by *Burkholderia cepacia* from contaminated intravenous flush solutions prepared by a compounding pharmacy in another state. *Pediatrics* 118(1): 212–5

Ho KM., Litton E (2006) Use of chlorhexidine-impregnated dressing to prevent vascular and epidural catheter colonization and infection: A meta-analysis. *Journal of Antimicrobial Chemotherapy* 58: 281–7

Jackson A (1998) Infection control: A battle in vein infusion phlebitis. *Nursing Times* 94(4): 68–71

Jackson A (2007) Development of a trust-wide vascular access team. *Nursing Times* 103(44): 28–9

Johnson JR, Kuskowski MA, Wilt TJ (2006) Systematic review: Antimicrobial urinary catheters to prevent catheter-associated urinary tract infection in hospitalised patients. *Annals of Internal Medicine* 144(2): 116–26

Kunin CM, McCormack RC (1966) Prevention of catheter-induced urinary tract infections by sterile closed drainage. *New England Journal of Medicine* 274(21): 1155–61

Kurladze GV (2007) *Environmental microbiology research trends.* Nova Science, New York

Maki DG, Ringer M, Alvarado CJ (1991) Prospective randomized trial of povidone-iodine, alcohol and chlorhexidine for prevention of infection associated with central venous and arterial catheters. *Lancet* **338**: 339–43

Maki DG, Tambyah PA (2001) Engineering out the risk of infection with urinary catheters. *Emerging Infectious Diseases* **7**(2): 342–7

Maki DG, Stolz SM, Wheeler S, Mermel LA (1997) Prevention of central venous catheter-related bloodstream infection by use of an antiseptic-impregnated catheter. A randomized, controlled trial. *Annals of Internal Medicine* **127**(4): 257–66

Mattner F, Gastmeier P (2004) Bacterial contamination of multiple-dose vials: A prevalence study. *American Journal of Infection Control* **32**(1): 12–16

Nacey JN, Tulloch AG, Ferguson AF (1985) Catheter-induced urethritis: A comparison between latex and silicone catheters in a prospective clinical trial. *British Journal of Urology* **57**: 325–8

Nazarko L (2008) Reducing the risk of catheter related urinary tract infection. *British Journal of Nursing* **17**(16): 1002–6

Nazarko L (2009) Providing effective evidence-based catheter management. British *Journal of Nursing (Continnence supplement)* **18**(7): S4–S12

Palefski SS, Stoddard GJ (2001) The infusion nurse and patient complication rates of peripheral-short catheters. A prospective evaluation. *Journal of Intravenous Nursing* **24**(2): 113–23

Pittet D, Tarara D, Wenzel RP (1994) Nosocomial bloodstream infection in critically ill patients. Excess length of stay, extra costs, and attributable mortality. *Journal of the American Medical Association* **271**(20): 1598–601

Pratt RJ, Pellowe CM, Wilson JA, Loveday HP, et al (2007) Epic2: National evidence based guidelines for preventing healthcare associated infections in NHS hospitals in England. *Journal of Hospital Infection* **65**: S1–S64

Raad I, Fang X, Keutgen XM, Jiang Y, Shertz R, Hachem R (2008) The role of chelators in preventing biofilm formation and catheter related bloodstream infections. *Current Opinion in Infectious Disease* **21**(4): 385–92

Rao GG, Elliot TSJ (1988) Bladder irrigation. *Age and Ageing* **17**: 373–8

Rickard CM, Vannapraseuth B, McGrail MR, Keene LJ, Rambaldo S, Smith CA, Ray-Barruel G (2009) The relationship between intravenous infusate colonisation and fluid container hang time. *Journal of Clinical Nursing* **18**(21): 3022–8

Royal College of Nursing (2010) *Standards for infusion therapy* (3rd edn) Royal College of Nursing, London

Robinson J (2006) Selecting a urinary catheter drainage system. *British Journal of Nursing* **15**(19): 1045–50

Saint S, Chenoweth CE (2003) Biofilms and catheter associated urinary tract infections. *Infectious Diseases North America* **17**(2): 411–32

Schears GJ (2006) Summary of product trials for 10,164 patients: Comparing an intravenous stabilizing device to tape. *Journal of Infusion Nursing* **29**(4): 225–31

Schumm K, Lam TB (2008) Types of urethral catheters for management of short term voiding problems in hospitalised adults: A short version. *Cochrane review Neurology and Neurodynamics* **27**(8): 738Cochrane review Neurourol urodyn46

Seymou VM, Dhallu TS, Mos HA, Tebb SE, Elliot TSJ (2000) A prospective clinical study to investigate the microbial contamination of a needleless connector. *Journal of Hospital Infection* **45**(2): 165–8

Soiffer E, Borzak A, Brian R, Weinstein RA (1998) Prevention of peripheral venous catheter complications with an intravenous therapy team: Randomised trial. *Journal of Internal Medicine* **158**: 473–7

Srinivasan A, Karchmer T, Richards A, Song X, Perl TM (2006) A prospective trial of a novel silicone-based silver coated foley catheter for the prevention of nosocomial urinary tract infections. *Infection Control and Hospital Epidemiology* **27**(1): 38–43

Tambyah PA, Maki DG (2000) Catheter-associated urinary tract infection is rarely symptomatic: A prospective study of 1,497 catheterized patients. *Archives of Internal Medicine* **160**(5): 678–82

Tindall AJ, Shetty AA, Rand C (2002) An unusual case of a postoperative bone cyst. *Journal of Bone and Joint Surgery* (British volume) **84**(6): 897–8

Ward V, Wilson J, Taylor L, Cookson B, Glynn A (1997) *Preventing hospital acquired infection: Clinical guidelines.* Public Health Laboratory Service, London

Webster J, Osborne S, Rickard C, Hall J (2010) Clinically-indicated replacement versus routine replacement of peripheral venous catheters. *Cochrane Database Systematic Reviews* **17**(3): CD007798

World Health Organization (2009) *WHO guidelines on hand hygiene in health care.* World Health Organization, Geneva

Woodward S (2005) Use of lubricant in female urethral catheterization. *British Journal of Nursing* **14**(19): 1022–23

CHAPTER 10

Caring for an infected patient

Rachel Ben Salem

Purpose

The purpose of this chapter is to provide an overview of the general principles of caring for an infected patient. It builds on the previous chapters and highlights specific areas for consideration.

Learning outcomes

By the end of the chapter, you will have learned:

- The challenges around healthcare-associated infections.
- The various issues to consider when caring for an infected patient.
- The care of patients with specific infections.
- How to prevent the spread of infection to others.

Introduction

Infectious diseases can occur in any setting, such as in patients' homes, in care homes and institutions and in hospitals. As a result, treatment and care of patients may take place across different types of residential care settings (including patients' homes) and in different specialist clinical areas, such as surgical wards, medical wards, intensive care units, coronary care units, and care of the elderly wards.

Preventing patients acquiring infections is the best policy; therefore, all healthcare workers have to be skilled in preventing the complications and spread of infections.

Prevalence of infections

The prevalence rate of infection is the proportion of a defined group of people that has an infection at any one point of time (Ayliffe et al 2000).

In the first two national infection prevalence surveys in UK hospitals (1980 and 1994) (Emmerson et al 1996), the rate of infection was 9.0% (equivalent to at least 300 000 healthcare-associated infections per year). In the third prevalence survey conducted in 2006 (Hospital Infection Society and Infection Control Nurses Association 2006), 8.2% of adult patients in acute hospitals were found to have a healthcare-associated infection. A Scottish survey in 2007 (Reilly et al 2007) gives an estimate of 9.5%. The aim of these prevalence surveys was to ascertain the number of patients in hospital who had or were being treated for an infection that they did not have on admission. In the third prevalence survey carried out in 2006 the commonest infections were:

*   Gastrointestinal system (22.0%).
*   Urinary tract (19.7%).
*   Pneumonia (13.9%).
*   Surgical site (13.8%).

As seen above, the gastrointestinal and urinary systems are the most common places for patients to develop an infection.

Incubation periods for infectious diseases

Incubation periods describe the time taken from when a person is exposed to the infectious disease to when they start to develop symptoms. The time may vary depending on the nature of the pathogen. Some diseases are more communicable during the incubation period than during the actual illness (e.g. hepatitis A, measles), therefore there is a high risk of cross-infection during that period. The mode of transmission and prevention of spread has already been discussed in previous chapters, and the reader is recommended to revisit these chapters for further information.

Special factors to consider

Age

When considering how best to care for patients with infections, it is important to note the patient's age. Children and elderly people are less able to resist infections and are more vulnerable because of either an immature or old and waning immune system. This needs to be taken into consideration when caring for clients within these age groups.

Surveillance

In addition, it is useful to be aware of where the patient was when they acquired the infection (i.e. developed the symptoms), or where the specimen was sent from, as this information will help with the surveillance of infections and the taking of appropriate and necessary action. For instance, patients may acquire an infection at home (nosohusial) and bring the infection into hospital with them, or may acquire it within the hospital environment (nosocomial).

It is imperative to follow MRSA screening policies on admission and during continuing care. The healthcare organisation's operational manager needs to have a clear protocol for the use of siderooms and comply with the prioritisation of infectious diseases so that patients and relatives are not put at risk due to the inappropriate or poor allocation of siderooms.

Assessment of infection

In order to determine if a patient has an infection, investigations are required. Diagnostic samples to be examined include blood, stool, sputum, cerebrospinal fluid and urine. Other investigations may include chest x-rays, biopsies and swabs.

Treatment of patients with infections also includes clinical assessment of how patients are, whether or not they need ventilator or respiratory support, and whether or not they are cardiovascularly and haemodynamically stable. This will dictate whether they are nursed in a high dependency or monitored bed. Wherever the patient is nursed, the principles of risk assessment must be applied, i.e. what is the suspected organism, what is the route of transfer, and is it safe to use contact precautions with the patient in the main bay or does he or she need to be in a sideroom? The infection prevention and control team of the healthcare organisation can help with this assessment.

General principles of treatment

Your patient will depend on you and the rest of the team for physical, social, spiritual and psychological support. This may include hygiene, nutrition and elimination. The level of support the patient requires will vary from patient to patient and can range from minimal support to total patient care.

Patients with infections tend to have a higher than normal temperature and this may lead to a fever. In the early stages of a fever, the patient often feels cold and starts to shiver. This is the body's response to a rising temperature –

the blood vessels in your skin constrict to conserve heat and maintain blood flow to the internal organs. The outer skin layer then becomes cool and your muscles start to contract. This makes you shiver. The body then responds by cooling down using evaporation and sweating. The very young and elderly are more likely to get complications from a fever. In the elderly, the part of the brain that regulates temperature (the hypothalamus) does not work as well as it does in the young. The body temperature can rise too much, causing heart problems and confusion. Young children may also have a convulsion (seizure) if their temperature gets too high.

Treatment of fever

A high temperature may be relieved by a damp cool flannel, and bed covers can be pulled back leaving just a sheet covering the patient. Regular changing of sheets and frequent turning of the pillows may aid comfort in patients who are perspiring. Use of paracetamol may also reduce temperature but careful dosing and temperature monitoring should be noted when antipyretics are used.

Fans are not suitable for a healthcare environment; they do not cool the patient particularly well and may spread air-borne pathogens throughout the healthcare environment.

Nutrition and hydration

Nursing patients with infections is aimed at helping them to fight the infection through their own host defences. A diet high in protein and vitamins supports the immune system in the formation of antibodies. Rehydration is vital where patients have high temperatures and excessive perspiration, or have excessive fluid loss through copious diarrhoea. Frequent drinks are needed in patients who have a high temperature or a dry or coated mouth. Furthermore, fluids will help dilute and excrete toxins from the body. A member of the medical team will be able to advise on specific electrolyte replacement as this too may be needed during an infection.

Reassurance and rest

Patients may suffer from anxiety, fear and apprehension (Watson 1979), which can be exacerbated when they are informed they have an infection. Generally, the more healthcare workers keep patients informed about treatment and procedures, the more likely their anxieties will be reduced.

Key points

When looking after patients with infections consider the following:
* Age
* Temperature
* Need for hydration and nutrition
* Support with aspects of care, such as personal hygiene
* Rest
* Reassurance
* Support from other specialists

During hospitalisation it is very important that patients are given time to ask questions about suspected and confirmed infections and are reassured and responded to. If the patient has a specific infection, then, where possible, the relevant specialist should be involved in providing support and information, e.g. if the patient has tuberculosis (TB) then the TB nurse specialist would be a key resource for information and reassurance. It is important that student nurses and others looking after patients are well-informed about infections and their implications and are ready to provide explanations to patients and relatives.

All patients need adequate rest so that they can heal, combat infection and recover. Nursing care should be coordinated so that the patient receives minimal disturbance. However, if the patient is being nursed within a sideroom or bay, then regular checks are necessary as patients in siderooms often feel neglected and isolated. There may be other psychological implications to being nursed in a sideroom, such as anxiety, fear and depression (Davies and Rees 2000).

Standard precautions

As mentioned in previous chapters, safe working practices include not putting patients or staff, including yourself, at risk of infection. Therefore the principles of standard precautions are necessary. These should be applied regardless of whether or not the patient is infectious. It is important to note that not all patients with an infectious disease will be symptomatic, neither may infection be the reason for their admission to hospital. Staff must remind themselves of all the safety elements, including:

185

- Hand hygiene.
- Appropriate use of gloves and aprons.
- Blood and body fluid precautions.
- Correct use of disinfectants.
- Aseptic technique.
- Disposal of sharps, waste and linen.
- Isolation precautions when patients have a known or suspected transmissible infection.

Contact precautions (or bedside isolation)

When a patient is being nursed with contact precautions, it is essential to have non-sterile disposable gloves and aprons available for use, and ensure these are worn appropriately and disposed of correctly to prevent cross-infection to other patients. All staff and relatives must be aware the patient is being nursed with contact precautions and be taught how to comply. Ideally, the patient should be in a sideroom, or near a clinical hand wash basin and foot-operated waste bin. Alcohol hand rub should be accessible at the point of patient care (although note that alcohol hand rub does not kill *Clostridium difficile* spores and only hand washing will suffice). Patients with suspected transmissible and confirmed diarrhoeal/vomiting diseases or open pulmonary TB must be in a sideroom with en suite toilet and bathroom. Negative pressure ventilation must be used for patients with suspected or confirmed open pulmonary TB.

Personal protective equipment (PPE) (as mentioned in previous chapters, this includes gloves, apron, mask, goggles and gowns) are designed to protect staff and others in healthcare settings from exposure to potentially infectious material. When providing care to patients, these products protect the skin and mucous membranes of the eyes, nose, and mouth from exposure to blood, body and respiratory secretions. Always perform hand hygiene immediately before applying and after removing PPE. Always apply PPE before contact with patients.

Wound infections

In some cases infection is due to an infected wound or to the patient's physical condition, and there may be a risk of developing pressure ulcers if due care is not taken to monitor and prevent this. A wound is a breach in the patient's skin integrity and as such presents a risk of infection.

It is especially important on admission and regularly afterwards to check the integrity of the patient's skin and document and manage wounds as part of the patient's care. Wounds can become contaminated with microorganisms that may cause an infection and delay wound healing.

Wounds occur for many different reasons including surgery; increased pressure; diseases such as diabetes; medications, e.g. steroids; circulation problems; and other problems, including burns. The aim in the treatment of wounds is to get them healed. The presence of a wound may change body image as well as lead to changes in lifestyle. It is important that the principles of asepsis (no touch technique) are applied to wounds to prevent cross-infection from the environment to the wound and vice versa. Furthermore, it is important that patients who are unable to change their positions regularly are assisted with this to prevent pressure ulcer formation; the tissue viability nurse is a good resource to refer patients to, and for advice.

Antibiotics

Sometimes, in addition to host defences, antibiotics are necessary to kill microorganisms, as in the management of acute bacterial infections. However at other times the immune system may be able to cope on its own. The next chapter provides an in-depth look at antimicrobials.

Policies and guidelines

It is a necessity to have policies and guidelines on how to avoid the spread of infection. Burnet and White (1972) chart the natural history of infectious diseases, which can help further understanding of the changing trends in disease and infection. Since the emergence of MRSA and other antibiotic-resistant organisms and the Stanley Royd Hospital outbreak of *Salmonella*, infection control policies have been produced.

The Health and Social Care Act 2008, which superseded the Hygiene Code 2006, requires all trusts to have clear arrangements for the effective prevention, detection and control of healthcare-associated infections, including MRSA, respiratory illness, diarrhoeal outbreaks, *Clostridium difficile* infection and transmissible spongiform encephalopathies, and the procedures to be taken in the event of an outbreak (Department of Health 2009).

Healthcare workers need to be familiar with these procedures and the relevant treatments. It is common practice for random audits to be carried out by healthcare organisations to ensure staff are working in line with the policies and procedures and are not placing clients/patients at undue risk.

Care of patients with specific infections

Infective diarrhoea

A visual guide has been developed describing the different types of stool (Bristol Stool Form) (Saad et al 2010). This grades the types of stool passed from hard nuts (type 1) through to a liquid stool (type 7). Types 1 and 2 indicate constipation; types 3 and 4 being the 'ideal stools', especially the latter, as they are the easiest to defecate; and types 5–7 tending towards diarrhoea.

Patients with type 6 or 7 should have their stool outputs monitored on a stool chart during the duration of passing liquid stools. It is also necessary to describe the frequency and document whether stool samples have already been sent to the laboratory for investigation. Stool specimens should be sent to microbiology for culture and sensitivity and to test for *C. difficile*. During times of increased incidence of norovirus and other common gastrointestinal viral infections including rotavirus, stools should be sent to virology. Check what your local infection control policy advises. Patients with frequent motions may become

---

Case study

Your hospital has seen a rise in the number of cases of norovirus and wards have been closed in response.

Patient Y develops liquid stool twice overnight. On checking, no stools have been sent to virology or microbiology for testing. Patient Y is very anxious and depressed regarding her recent diagnosis of cancer and does not want to be moved into a sideroom. The infection control nurse later in the day confirms that the patient Y is *Clostridium difficile* positive. Patient Y still refuses to go into the sideroom. The next day the patient has not moved and the infection control team come to review her. They advise isolation with en suite facilities and ask for patient Y's psychiatrist to come and review her. During the meeting the infection control nurse is informed that the patient Y is also norovirus positive. The patient still refuses to go into the sideroom.

Consider the scenario and decide the best course of action you can take to address each of the challenges that arise when looking after patient Y. Where possible, refer to your organisation's policies and guidelines for further information.

---

dehydrated and therefore should be managed on a fluid balance chart noting fluids in and out. Nurses who look after patients with liquid stools or diarrhoea need to ensure that patients are aware that their stool motions need to be recorded. Also, patients with suspected or confirmed infectious diarrhoea, including *Clostridium difficile*, norovirus, etc., will need to be nursed in a sideroom with en suite toilet facilities, or given their own commode. This is to prevent cross-infection to other patients. Toilets and commodes should be cleaned carefully after use and should be subject to infection control and environmental cleaning audits.

In addition to the care provided to the patient with infective diarrhoea, patients with suspected *Clostridium difficile* will require isolation in a sideroom if they have had two episodes of diarrhoea whilst receiving antibiotics. Furthermore, in some cases, further investigation may be required to assess the extent of the disease. This may include colonoscopy or sigmoidoscopy where a camera is inserted into the colon with a biopsy being taken during the procedure when necessary.

Open pulmonary TB

Patients with suspected open pulmonary TB may be investigated with a chest x-ray and three sputum samples. Samples should be collected and sent to microbiology for TB testing. A blood test can be taken from asymptomatic people where TB disease may be latent. Patients may also have a bronchoscopy if they are not coughing. At every step of the way the patient should be kept informed of what is happening and prepared for future procedures and treatment.

Patients should not wear a surgical filter mask in a sideroom for infection control purposes. The only time patients should wear an appropriate mask is when they are transferring between siderooms or for necessary investigations. A patient with suspected or confirmed TB should then wear a surgical mask. Surgical masks are designed to prevent the respiratory secretions of the person wearing the mask from entering the air.

Patients may require bronchoscopy, a procedure where a flexible or sometimes rigid scope is passed into the lungs via the nose or mouth and the endoscopist takes pictures and, where necessary, a biopsy of tissue.

MRSA-positive patients

MRSA may affect patients at any point of hospitalisation. A patient may be colonised with MRSA, e.g. it is present on the skin, in the nostrils or another area of the body. However, this does not mean the patient has an infection. The

---

Stop, check, ask...

- Do you know where the following policies are:
  - MRSA policy
  - *Clostridium difficile* policy
  - Infection control policy?
- Have you recently received training on any of the policies or procedures you undertake, e.g. hand washing aseptic technique, use of PPE?
- Do your know how to contact your infection prevention and control team?

---

healthcare worker must be able to distinguish between the two states, and explain this to the patient in order to allay anxiety. Patients may be colonised with MRSA on admission and may be unaware of this. Therefore, all patients admitted to the healthcare setting are screened according to local MRSA policy, and results are followed up by clinical teams. Always check that patients have been screened, what the result is, and when they should be screened again.

Patients colonised with MRSA need to be managed as MRSA positive and must be nursed with contact precautions. Most patients will be prescribed MRSA suppression treatment according to local policy.

The suppression treatment usually includes a nasal cream to be applied to both nostrils three to four times a day and a daily body wash which includes washing of the hair. The local protocol should be followed.

It is important to help the patient by maintaining good hygiene, including clean hands at all times, as well as maintaining a clean environment. It is also important that patients are reassured that MRSA is treatable and that an MRSA positive result (e.g. being colonised with MRSA) does not automatically mean that they have an infection. However, patients must be monitored for signs and symptoms of infection.

Most acute hospitals will isolate a patient with MRSA, since, if they are nursed in an open bay, it is difficult to control spread to other susceptible patients, i.e. those who have surgical wounds, urinary catheters, intravenous lines and pressure sores. However, where it is not possible to practise this, e.g. due to insufficient siderooms, strict infection control procedures should be followed. Please refer to local infection control policies and prioritisation of siderooms lists.

When providing care to patients with any type of infection it is important to make relevant patient information leaflets available as these will help to reinforce any messages provided to the patient.

Summary

In this chapter we have looked at the various aspects of care required for patients who have acquired an infection. The benefits of prevalence studies in helping to identify the extent of infections has been briefly discussed. The chapter has also examined three specific infections that are common within most healthcare settings, and how best to care for patients with them.

The next chapter will look in detail at one of the most important aspects of care when preventing or treating an infected patient – the use of antimicrobials.

References

Ayliffe G, Fraise A, Geddes A, Mitchell K (2000) *Control of hospital infection. A practical handbook* (4th edn) Arnold Hodder, LondonBiology-online.org (2008) *Pathway of fever development in response to infection.* Available at: http://www.biology-online. org/articles/cytokine_regulation_fever_studies/figures.html [Accessed 17 August 10]

Burnet M, White D (1972) *Natural history of infectious disease.* Cambridge University Press, Cambridge

Davies H, Rees J (2000) Psychological effects of isolation nursing. (1) Mood disturbance. *Nursing Standard* **14**(28): 35–8

Department of Health (2009) *Health and Social Care Act 2008: Code of Practice for health and adult social care on the prevention and control of infections and related guidance.* Department of Health, London

Emmerson AM, Enstone JE, Griffin M, Kelsey MC, Smyth ET (1996) The Second National Prevalence Survey of Infection in Hospitals. Overview of the results. *Journal of Hospital Infection* **32**(2): 175–90

Hospital Infection Society and Infection Control Nurses Association (2006) *Third Prevalence Survey of Healthcare Associated Infections in Acute Hospitals 2006: Summary of preliminary results.* Hospital Infection Society and Infection Control Nurses Association, London

Reilly J, Stewart S, Allardice G, Noone A, Robertson C, Walker A (2007) *NHS Scotland National HAI Prevalence Survey: Final report.* Health Protection Scotland, Edinburgh

Saad R, Rao S, Koch K, Kuo B, Parkman H, McCallum R, Sitrin M, Wilding G Semler J, Chey W (2010) Do stool form and frequency correlate with whole-gut and colonic transit? Results from a multicenter study. *American Journal of Gastroenterology* **105**(2): 403–11

Watson J (1979) *Medical-surgical nursing and related physiology*. McMillan, Houndsmill, Basingstoke

Further reading

Burnet M, White D (1972) *The natural history of infectious diseases*. Cambridge University Press, Cambridge

CHAPTER 11

Antibacterial agents and their role in infection control

Christianne Micallef

Purpose

The purpose of this chapter is to provide an overview of the various types of antibacterial agents and their actions. The chapter then examines the general principles of safe prescribing and the use of antibacterial agents.

Learning outcomes

By the end of the chapter, you will have learned:

- The historical perspective of infectious disease and its impact on the development of antibacterial agents.
- Commonly used antibacterial agents and how they work.
- Best practice around the use of antibacterial agents.
- An overview of resistance to antibiotics.

Introduction

In England, the Health and Social Care Act 2008 Code of Practice (Department of Health 2009) for health and adult social care on the prevention and control of infections and related guidance is currently used in order to certify that a healthcare institution has procedures in place to prevent and control healthcare-associated infections (HCAIs). This document also specifies the need for local evidence-based antimicrobial guidelines as well as an antimicrobial stewardship strategy, which includes audits.

Key strategies to ensure antimicrobial stewardship include the establishment of an antimicrobial management team, which should include a medical microbiologist and an antimicrobial pharmacist. This chapter will look at this in further detail.

Historical perspective on infectious diseases and the advent of chemotherapeutic agents

In the late 18th century, the pioneering of smallpox vaccine by Edward Jenner marked the beginning of chemotherapy for infectious diseases and the eventual declaration in 1978 that smallpox had been eradicated. In the 19th century, Louis Pasteur developed vaccines against anthrax, cholera and rabies (Frankland and Frankland 1901). The development of agents that were effective in the treatment of bacterial infections took much longer.

The fight against bacterial diseases began in the early 20th century with the isolation and identification of *Treponema pallidum*, the causative agent of syphilis, by Eric Hoffman and Fritz Schaudinn. This was followed in 1906 by the development of a diagnostic blood test for antibodies to syphilis by August von Wassermann. In 1910, Paul Ehrlich, the father of antimicrobial chemotherapy, created Salvarsan (arsphenamine), an arsenic derivative, which was hailed a 'magic bullet'. Arsphenamine proved to be toxic and quite difficult to administer. In 1912, Neosalvarsan (neoarsphenamine) was developed. Although less toxic and more soluble than the parent compound, it was also less effective (Greenwood et al 2008). It was not until the late 1920s that the development of true antibiotics really began. In 1929, Alexander Fleming published his discovery of penicillin, but the importance of this was not recognised until the 1940s. Prontosil, the first sulphonamide, was developed by the German chemist Gerhard Domagk from a red azo dye which was found to have antibacterial activity against the Gram-positive bacteria *Staphylococcus* and *Streptococcus*. In 1939 Howard Florey and Ernst Chain

---

Antibacterial agents: Timeline

- Late 18th century: Smallpox vaccine by Edward Jenner
- 19th century: Vaccines against anthrax, cholera, rabies developed by Louis Pasteur
- 1929: Penicillin discovered by Alexander Fleming
- 1940s: Prontosil discovered by Gerhard Domagk
- 1943: *Penicillin chysogenum* discovered by Mary Hunt, enabling large-scale production of penicillin
- 1943: Streptomycin discovered by Selman Waksman, Albert Schatz and Elizabeth Bugie

---

began their research into penicillin and in 1943, Mary Hunt discovered *Penicillin chysogenum,* the catalyst enabling the mass production of penicillin as an antibiotic, which was marketed in 1945. It was also in 1943 that Selman Waksman, Albert Schatz and Elizabeth Bugie discovered streptomycin, the first aminoglycoside, a naturally occurring antibiotic synthesised by the soil organism *Streptomyces griseus,* which became instrumental in the treatment of tuberculosis.

The era of antibiotics had truly begun, and in 1967 William Stewart, the US Surgeon General, made the statement that infectious diseases had been conquered. We now know that this was a premature belief. Today, the activity of many classes of antibiotics is being threatened by resistance. Mortality and morbidity from infectious diseases has changed very little since the beginning of the 20th century. In 2009, the World Health Organization's World Health Statistics estimated that, despite the development of effective vaccines and numerous classes of antibiotics, infectious diseases were responsible for more than 30% of neonatal deaths and 51% of years of life lost globally (WHO 2009). The search for new and effective antibiotics continues. Recently, the Infectious Diseases Society of America (IDSA) launched its '10 by 20' initiative to develop 10 new, safe and effective antibiotics by 2020 (IDSA, 2010). The success of this initiative may be vital if we are to be able to treat bacterial infections with effective agents in the coming decades.

Mode of action of antibacterial agents

Currently, a number of antibacterial agents are available for clinical use; the mode of action of some common examples are given in *Table 11.1.*

In the following section we will look at some of the most commonly used agents.

Properties and activities of selected antibacterial agents

Penicillins

Pencillin G

This is a natural occurring penicillin that was originally produced from *Penicillium* spp.

Issues of administration: Penicillin G is inactivated by gastric acid and can only be used parenterally, i.e. intravenously.

Table 11.1. Antibacterial agents and their modes of action

Antibacterial class and examples	Mode of action	Clinical indications
Sulphonamides: • sulphamethoxazole, trimethoprim	• Inhibition of bacterial metabolic pathways	• *Pneumocystis jirovecii* pneumonia, nocardiosis, toxoplasmosis
Aminoglycosides: • streptomycin, gentamicin, netilmicin, tobramycin, amikacin	• Inhibition of initiation complex in bacterial protein synthesis	• Abdominal infections • Serious infections, e.g. endocarditis (often used in combination with penicillins)
Penicillins: (beta-lacatam) • penicillin G (benzylpenicillin) • penicillin V (phenoxymethylpenicillin) • flucloxacillin, amoxicillin, piperacillin, ticarcillin	• Inhibition of bacterial cell wall cross-linking by targeting penicillin-binding proteins (PBPs)	• Respiratory tract infections • Cellulitis • Urinary tract infections
Cephalosporins: (beta-lacatam) • cephradine, cephalexin cefpodoxil, cefuroxime, cefotaxime, ceftriaxone, cefepime	• Inhibition of bacterial cell wall cross-linking by targeting PBPs	• Respiratory tract infections • Urinary tract infections • Cellulitis
Carbapenems: (beta-lacatam) • imipenem, meropenem, ertapenem, doripenem	• Inhibition of bacterial cell wall cross-linking by targeting PBPs	• Life-threatening infections typically unresponsive to other first-line agents
Monobactams: (beta-lacatam) • aztreonam	• Inhibition of bacterial cell wall cross-linking by targeting PBPs	• Gram-negative infections often unresponsive to previous therapy
Glycopeptides: • vancomycin, teicoplanin	• Act on the precursors of bacterial cell wall synthesis	• Serious staphylococcal infections. Vancomycin is given orally for *Clostridium difficile* infection

Tetracyclines: • oxytetracycline, minocycline, doxycycline	• Inhibition of aminoacyl-containing end of tRNA from binding to the mRNA in bacterial protein synthesis-elongation step	• Respiratory tract infections • Sexually transmitted diseases (STDs)
Macrolides: • erythromycin, clarithromycin, azithromycin	• Inhibition of translocation step in bacterial protein synthesis-translation step	• Respiratory tract infections • Cellulitis • STDs
Streptogramin: • quinupristin/dalfopristin	• Inhibition of bacterial protein synthesis	• Serious Gram-positive infections, generally unresponsive to other antibiotics
Cyclic lipopeptide: • daptomycin	• Termination of bacterial DNA, RNA and protein synthesis	• Serious staphylococal infections, unresponsive to other antibiotics
Glycylcyclines: • tigeycycline	• Inhibition of aminoacyl-containing end of tRNA from binding to the mRNA in bacterial protein synthesis-elongation step	• Skin and soft tissue infections • Complicated abdominal infections
Rifamycin: • rifampicin	• Inhibits bacterial RNA polymerase and hence RNA synthesis	• Tuberculosis • Used as adjunct to treat serious staphylococcal infections
Fluoroquinolones: • nalidixic acid, norfloxacin, ofloxacin, ciprofloxacin, levofloxacin, moxifloxacin	• Inhibit bacterial DNA replication	• Gram-negative infections • Newer fluroquinolones (e.g. levofloxacin and moxifloxacin) have enhanced activity against drug-resistant pneumococcal infections
5-Nitroimidazole: • metronidazole	• Acts on bacterial DNA	• Anaerobic infections (has antiparasitic activity)

Clinical indications: Benzylpenicillin is used for the treatment of pneumococcal pneumonia, endocarditis, anthrax, cellulitis and meningococcal disease.

Spectrum of use: The spectrum of Penicillin G includes penicillin-susceptible *Staphylococcus aureus*, streptococci, *Neisseria* spp., anaerobic cocci, *Clostridium* spp., *Pasteurella multocida, Fusobacterium* spp., *Prevotella* spp. and *Porphyromonas* spp. (Murray et al 2007).

Penicillin V

This is also a natural occurring penicillin originally produced from *Penicillium* spp.

Issues of administration: Penicillin V is gastric-acid stable therefore can be administered orally.

Clinical indications: Main indications include treatment of tonsillitis, otitis media, erysipelas and cellulitis.

Spectrum of use: It has a similar antibacterial spectrum to Penicillin G, although it is less effective against *N. gonorrhoea*. Beta-lactamase-producing strains are resistant to both penicillin V and penicillin G (Hauser 2007, Royal Pharmaceutical Society 2010).

Flucloxacillin

Issues of administration: It is available as both oral and parenteral preparation. The oral preparation needs to be taken at least half an hour before food.

Clinical indications: Flucloxacillin uses include otitis externa, skin and soft tissue infections, osteomyelitis and endocarditis (due to staphylococci). Caution needs to be exercised if patients have hepatic disease, as this drug may cause cholestatic jaundice and kernicterus in neonates.

Spectrum of use: Flucloxacillin is a narrow-spectrum antibiotic, indicating that its activity is limited to penicillinase-producing and non-penicillinase-producing staphylococci as well as streptococci, gonococci, meningococci and Gram-positive anaerobes (Finch et al 2003).

Amoxicillin

Issues of administration: This agent can be administered both orally and intravenously.

Clinical indications: It is used for treatment of pneumonia, otitis media, anthrax, urinary tract infections, *Listeria* spp. meningitis and endocarditis.

Spectrum of use: Amoxicillin is a broad-spectrum aminopenicillin with activity similar to penicillin G but is active against enterococci and *Listeria* spp.

Extended-spectrum penicillins

The extended-spectrum penicillins (Esps), include the ureidopenicillins, such as piperacillin, and carboxypenicillins, such as ticarcillin.

Co-amoxiclav (amoxicillin plus the beta-lactamase inhibitor clavulanic acid) is indicated if strains produce β-lactamases, although clavulanic acid does not inhibit class D β-lactamases or class B metallo-β-lactamases, and indeed may induce the production of these enzymes in some bacteria. Both compounds may cause cholestatic jaundice and should be avoided in patients predisposed to this condition. This risk is much higher with co-amoxiclav, than with amoxicillin

The extended-spectrum penicillins have improved Gram-negative activity, including *Pseudomonas* spp. These include piperacillin and ticarcillin.

Issues of administration: These are given intravenously.

Clinical indications: Extended-spectrum penicillins are indicated for moderate to severe infections including bloodstream infections.

Spectrum of use: They are active against anaerobes (e.g. *Bacteroides fragilis*) and have Gram-positive activity (e.g. staphylococci). Piperacillin is also available with the β-lactamase inhibitor tazobactam and has better activity against *P. aeruginosa* than ticarcillin.

Reaction to penicillins

Hypersensitivity reactions may occur with the administration of all penicillins. This ranges from 1–10% of all treated patients (Royal Pharmaceutical Society 2010). Patients who develop a slight rash may be treated with other β-lactam antibiotics, such as cephalosporins and carbapenems. In patients who have a history of an anaphylactic type of reaction, all β-lactam antibiotics should be avoided.

Typical common side-effects of penicillins include gastrointestinal upset. Rarely, blood dyscrasias (e.g. thrombocytopenia, haemolytic anaemia, etc.) may occur. Penicillins are primarily excreted renally and, in patients with renal dysfunction require dose modification according to the patient's creatinine clearance (Murray et al 2007).

Table 11.2 provides a summary of bacteria susceptible to different pencillins.

Cephalosporins

Another group of β-lactam antibiotics are the cephalosporins. These were

Table 11.2. Spectrum of activity of penicillins

Penicillin antibiotic	Common susceptible bacteria
Penicillin G (benzylpenicillin), penicillin V (phenoxymethylpenicillin)	Streptococci, *Neisseria* spp., *Clostridium* spp. (except *Clostridium difficile*)
Flucloxacillin	Streptococci (e.g. *Streptococcus pyogenes*) and staphylococci, e.g *Staphylococcus aureus*
Amoxicillin (plus clavulanate, as β-lactamase inhibitor, to produce co-amoxiclav)	Gram-positive and Gram-negative and some anaerobes. β-lactamase-producing strains inactivate amoxicillin, so for these, co-amoxiclav is used instead
Piperacillin (plus tazobactam), ticarcillin (plus clavulanate), temocillin	Expanded Gram-negative activity coliforms and *Pseudomonas aeruginosa* Gram-positive and anaerobic activity

originally isolated from *Cephalosporium acremonium*, a mould found in sewage, by Giuseppe Brotzu in the 1940s (Hauser 2007), although it took another two decades for the class to achieve clinical utility (Mandell et al 2009).

Issues of administration: Like the penicillins, cephalosporins are generally well tolerated and can be given orally and intravenously.

Clinical indications: This group of drugs is commonly used for a wide range of clinical conditions depending on generation, e.g. first- and second-generation cephalosporins tend to be employed for the treatment of respiratory and urinary tract infections. Third-, fourth- and, recently, also the fifth-generation cephalosporins, are indicated for more severe infections, such as meningitis and bloodstream infections. The fifth-generation cephalosporins, i.e ceftobiprole (Kisgen and Whitney 2008) and ceftaroline (Barton and MacGowan 2009) have anti-MRSA activity but are not currently available in the UK. The main side-effect is hypersensitivity, with 0.5–6.5% of patients allergic to penicillins, being also allergic to cephalosporins (Royal Pharmaceutical Society 2010). Gastrointestinal side-effects are also common with these drugs. These agents are also associated with a high-risk for the development of *C. difficile* infection (Paterson 2004, Dubberke et al 2008, Gerding et al 2008, Monaghan et al 2008, Wilcox et al 2008). Additional side-effects include hepatic disorders and blood dyscrasias.

Spectrum of use: The cephalopsorins are active against a wide variety of aerobic and anaerobic bacteria. The most widely accepted classification divides these compounds into five divisions or generations. The first-generation have predominantly Gram-positive activity, the second has enhanced activity against Gram-negatives. Third-generation cephalosporins exhibit markedly increased activity against Gram-negative bacilli (ceftazidime has enhanced activity against *Pseudomonas aeruginosa*), but for some, the Gram-positive activity is actually reduced. The fourth-generation has the broadest spectrum, covering Gram-positive cocci and Gram-negative bacilli. The third- and fourth-generation cephalosporins are also called extended-spectrum cephalosporins. The fifth-generation cephalosporins have activity against methicillin-resistant *Staphylococcus aureus* and enhanced activity against *Streptococcus pneumoniae* and *Enterococcus faecalis* (Barton and MacGowan 2009, Mandell et al 2009).

Table 11.3 presents a brief summary of different cephalosporins and typical bacterial spectrum.

Table 11.3. Cephalosporins and common susceptible bacteria

Generation	Examples	Common susceptible bacteria
First-generation	Cephalexin, cephradine	Staphylococci, streptococci and some Gram-negative bacteria, e.g. *Escherichia coli*
Second-generation	Cefuroxime	Same as for first-generation and also exhibit increased activity against aerobic and facultative Gram-negative bacteria; includes a pronounced activity against *Haemophilus influenzae* (even β-lactamase-producing strains)
Third-generation	Cefotaxime, ceftriaxone, ceftazidime	Gram-positive and Gram-negative activity; ceftazidime only used for *P. aeruginosa* but not for staphylococci
Fourth-generation	Cefepime	Gram-positive and Gram-negative activity and includes *P. aeruginosa*
Fifth-generation	Ceftobiprole, ceftaroline	Gram-positive and Gram-negative and anti-MRSA activity
Adapted from Hauser 2007, Murray et al 2007, Kisgen and Whitney 2008, Barton and MacGowan 2009, Mandell et al 2009, BNF 2010		

Carbapenems

Carbapenems have the broadest spectrum of the β-lactam class. The carbapenems include imipenem, meropenem, ertapenem and doripenem.

Issues of administration: These are given intravenously.

Clinical indications: These are regarded as the 'big guns' and generally reserved for the treatment of serious hospital-acquired infections, which are often polymicrobial and where other agents have failed. Infections that are treated with carbapenems include hospital-acquired pneumonia, intra-abdominal infections, complicated urinary-tract infections and skin and soft tissue infections. The carbapenems are generally well tolerated and have a side-effect profile that is similar to other β-lactam antibiotics.

Spectrum of use: They have Gram-positive, Gram-negative and anaerobic activity. Imipenem needs to be given in conjunction with cilastatin, as it is inactivated by renal dipeptidase I and cilastatin counteracts this enzyme, permitting the antibiotic to act. This drug is not indicated in the presence of central nervous system (CNS) disorders or for CNS infections. Meropenem, doripenem and imipenem have a similar spectrum of activity. Ertapenem has a long half-life and can be administered on a daily basis. It has no activity against *Pseudomonas* and *Acinetobacter* spp. (Royal Pharmaceutical Society 2010). Carbapenems are generally active against extended-spectrum β-lactamase (ESBL)-producing *Enterobacteriaceae*, although the emergence of *Klebsiella pneumoniae* carbapenemases threatens the clinical utility of this class of antibiotics.

Monobactams

Aztreonam is a monobactam that is a narrow-spectrum β-lactam anti-bacterial.

Issues of administration: Monobactams are given intravenously.

Clinical indications: Aztreonam is used only for infections caused by Gram-negative bacteria.

Spectrum of use: They are not active against Gram-positive and anaerobic bacteria. Side-effects are similar as with other β-lactams but patients who are hypersensitive to penicillin demonstrate lower hypersensitivity to aztreonam (Royal Pharmaceutical Society 2010). Aztreonam has a pronounced activity against aerobic Gram-negative bacteria, e.g. *Haemophilus influenzae, Neisseria meningitidis* and *Pseudomonas aeruginosa*.

Glycopeptides

The glycopeptides are a group of chemically complex compounds obtained originally from soil actinomycetes (Finch et al 2003). Glycopeptides include vancomycin and teicoplanin.

Issues of administration: Vancomycin and teicoplanin are administered intravenously. An important caution with vancomycin is the ability to produce red neck/man syndrome on rapid administration. This is consistent with the massive release of histamine from mast cells, hence imparting the characteristic red colour. Doses above 500mg should be given over 1 hour as an infusion and never as a bolus, with the rate of administration never exceeding 10mg/minute (Royal Pharmaceutical Society 2010).

Oral vancomycin is indicated for the treatment *C. difficile* infection, as it has a local action and very poor systemic absorption. The parenteral preparation is licensed to be administered as a solution where patients cannot take capsules. This solution can be mixed with orange juice to enhance palatability and hence compliance.

Clinical indications: Glycopeptides are very important agents in the antibacterial armamentarium. They are predominantly used to treat MRSA infections. They can be used instead of penicillins where serious penicillin allergy has been documented. Since the mid-1990s resistance to the glycopeptides has emerged. Vancomycin-resistant enterococci and *Staphylococcus aureus* with reduced susceptibility to vancomycin are being increasingly reported in the literature. In addition, the development of resistance during therapy, or minimum inhibitory concentration-creep, is also increasingly being reported. Side-effects of glycopeptides include gastrointestinal upset, rashes, lacrimation, and blood dyscrasias.

Vancomycin is potentially ototoxic and nephrotoxic. The risk of toxicity is reduced by therapeutic drug monitoring. Vancomycin is an acidic drug and can cause extravasation and phlebitis when given intravenously.

Unlike vancomycin, teicoplanin does not cause significant histamine release. Nephrotoxicity is uncommon, and when it does occur is not related to dose, plasma concentration or concomitant therapy with an aminoglycoside. Thrombocytopenia has been reported in patients with raised trough levels (~60 mg/l) (Finch et al 2003).

Spectrum of use: Their activity is essentially limited to Gram-positive organisms, notably staphylococci and streptococci (Finch et al 2003).

Fluoroquinolones

The quinolone group of antibacterials are totally synthetic compounds. Nalidixic acid is the parent compound of quinolone antibacterial agents. Ofloxacin and norfloxacin were also among the early members of this group.

Ciprofloxacin is a fluoroquinolone with broad Gram-negative activity.

Issues of administration: Ciprofloxacin is the only oral agent available for the treatment of *Pseudomonas aeruginosa* infections. It can also be given intravenously. Levofloxacin and ofloxacin are also available orally and intravenously. Moxifloxacin, norfloxacin and nalidixic acid are available orally only.

Clinical indications: Nalidixic acid was primarily used for the treatment of urinary tract infections (UTIs) but its use has diminished greatly. Ofloxacin and norfloxacin are also primarily used for the treatment of UTIs and sexually transmitted diseases (STDs), although ofloxacin is also used for other indications, such as prostatitis, gonorrhoea and pelvic inflammatory disease.

An important, though rare, side-effect of quinolones is tendon damage. This occurs within 48 hours of initiating therapy. Additional side-effects include gastrointestinal effects, rashes, sleep disturbances, blood disorders, hepatic and renal dysfunction, photosensitivity and neurological reactions. Quinolones may induce convulsions in patients with epilepsy or even without a history of convulsions. The concomitant administration of non-steroidal anti-inflammatory drugs (NSAIDs) may contribute to this. Quinolones should not be taken with divalent metal cations, e.g. calcium and iron salts, as their absorption is reduced (Royal Pharmaceutical Society 2010).

The quinolones are considered high-risk antibiotics for the development of *C. difficile* infection (Dubberke et al 2008, Monaghan et al 2008) and may be a

---

Key points

- *Penicillins:* used to treat a wide range of minor to severe infections
- *Carbapenems and monobactams:* used for serious life-threatening infections, often unresponsive to other antibiotics
- *Glycopeptides:* used for serious Gram-positive infections, including MRSA and *C. difficile* infection
- *Cephalosporins:* similar uses to penicillins, though these have a coverage of Gram-negative bacteria

risk factor for the acquisition of MRSA infections (Paterson 2004, Dancer 2008, Liebowitz and Blunt 2008, Tacconelli et al 2008).

Spectrum of use: The primary route of elimination is renal. Ciprofloxacin is a fluoroquinolone with broad Gram-negative activity. It is only moderately effective in infections caused by Gram-positive cocci. Ciprofloxacin should not be used for the treatment of known pneumococcal infections.

Newer fluoroquinolones, levofloxacin and moxifloxacin, were initially launched for the treatment of drug-resistant *Streptococcus pneumoniae* and have activity against the pneumococcus. They also have Gram-negative activity. In 2008, the European Medicines Agency issued a warning regarding the use of moxifloxacin, because of an association with fatal hepatic reactions.

Aminoglycosides

The aminoglycosides are comprised of a large group of naturally occurring or semi-synthetic polycatonic compounds (Finch et al 2003). The first aminoglycoside to be used clinically was streptomycin. It is still used in cases of drug-resistant tuberculosis, unresponsive to other antibiotics. Other aminoglycosides include gentamicin, amikacin and tobramycin, the most important of which in clinical use is gentamicin. All aminoglycosides require routine therapeutic drug monitoring, and renal function needs to be assessed prior to commencement of therapy. Aminoglycosides are excreted by glomerular filtration. Dose-reduction is essential in renal failure to avoid toxicity.

Issues of administration: The aminoglycosides are administerd parenterally and typically via the intravenous route since, given intramuscularly, they are very painful.

Clinical indications: Aminoglycosides are used for the treatment of serious Gram-negative infections and as an adjunct to other antibiotics, e.g. penicillins, due to their synergistic effects.

*Spectrum of use:*Aminoglycosides are active to different degrees against *S. aureus*, coagulase-negative staphylococci and *Corynebacterium* spp., but their activity against other Gram-positives, including streptococci, is limited. They are frequently used in combination with other antibiotics because of their synergistic interaction.

Nomograms are commonly employed to predict peak concentration (Cmax) (Nicolau et al 1995). Aminoglycosides are concentration-dependent antibiotics and can be administered on a high-dose, once daily basis, to produce a post-antibiotic effect (PAE). When given in combination with other agents to

> **Remember...**
>
> - Cephalosporins and quinolones are known to predispose to *C. difficile* and MRSA infections and a risk–benefit analysis needs to be conducted prior to initiating therapy
> - Quinolones may interact with other medications: They should not be co-administered with dairy products, vitamins, NSAIDs or anti-epileptics
> - Quinolones may have serious side-effects: If tenderness develops in limbs up to 48hrs after starting therapy, STOP it immediately

provide a synergistic effect, lower doses may be used. Aminoglycosides are oto- and nephrotoxic and can produce neuromuscular blockade. Due to their nephrotoxic potential, they should not be used with other nephrotoxic agents, such as loop diuretics and glycopeptides. Aminoglycosides are contraindicated in myasthenia gravis.

Tetracyclines

Tetracyclines and their synthetic derivatives and are derived from *Streptomyces* spp. (an organism found in soil).

Issues of administration: Tetracyclines are only available orally.

Clinical indications: The use of tetracyclines has significantly declined because of increased resistance and the development of better tolerated agents, although they are still utilised for the treatment of atypical infections, such as legionellosis, syphilis, epididymitis, plague and leptospirosis. More recently, they have been used as part of multi-drug regimens in the management of gastritis and peptic ulcer disease.

Tetracyclines may produce gastrointestinal upset and should not be taken with dairy products as they interact with calcium as well as other metal cations, e.g. iron. Also, these agents are contra-indicated in children less than 12 years of age in the United Kingdom (8 years in USA) as they produce yellowing of the teeth and skeletal deformities. Pregnant women should not be treated with these agents. In addition, the major side effect which led to the decline in the use of these agents was discolouration of teeth.

Spectrum of use: They are essentially broad-spectrum bacteriostatic agents, effective for the treatment of Gram-positive and some aerobic Gram-negative infections. They have activity against the spirochaetes, such as *T. pallidum* and *Borrelia burgdorferi*.

Glycylcyclines

Tigecycline is a glycylcycline, which is a synthetic derivative of the tetracyclines. These compounds were developed to circumvent the major mechanisms of resistance to the tetracyclines.

Issues of administration: Tigecycline is poorly absorbed orally and is only available as an intravenous infusion.

Clinical indications: Licensed indications include complicated skin and soft tissue infections, and complicated intra-abdominal infections. It is a suitable option in the treatment of nosocomial multi-resistant bacterial infections caused by organisms such as MRSA or glycopeptide-resistant enterococci.

The major side effect associated with the use of tigecycline is nausea and vomiting which may occur in up to 20% of patients. Acute pancreatitis may occur but is rare (Barton and MacGowan 2009). There is also a tendency for the prothrombin time (and activated partial thromboplastin time) to increase when tigecycline is administered, so special attention needs to be ensured in patients on concomitant anti-coagulant therapy

Spectrum of use: Tigecycline has Gram-positive, Gram-negative and anaerobic activity. However, *Pseudomonas, Proteus* spp. and some strains of *Corynebacterium jeikeium* are resistant.

Macrolides and ketolides

The macrolides are a large group of closely related antibiotics produced mostly by *Streptomyces* and related species. They include erythromycin, clarithromycin and azithromycin. Telithromycin is obtained by semi-synthesis of erythromycin A and is classified as a ketolide.

Issues of administration: Macrolides are generally safe drugs and can be administered both orally and parenterally, except telithromycin, which is only available orally.

Clinical indications: They are active against atypicals including *Chlamydiae, Mycoplasma* and *Rickettsiae* and a number of mycobacteria. These agents are widely used, particularly for respiratory infections. Erythromycin is the parent compound and is also used for skin infections and sexually transmitted diseases. Clarithromycin covers the same organisms but achieves higher tissue concentrations. All macrolides and ketolides may cause QT prolongation and should not be used where patients exhibit this condition. Macrolides also interact with a number of common medications, e.g. HMG-

CoA reductase inhibitors (commonly known as statins) and warfarin. Serious adverse reactions are rare. The exception is erythromycin estolate, which is hepatotoxic. Gastrointestinal side-effects are the most commonly reported adverse event and occur more frequently with erythromycin than other members of the class.

Spectrum of use: Their spectrum includes most Gram-positive organisms, *Neisseria* spp., *Haemophilus* spp., *Bordetella pertussis, Moraxella catarrhalis* and Gram-positive and Gram-negative anaerobes. Clarithromycin is normally given twice a day (12 hourly) whilst erythromycin is four times a day (6 hourly), which may be important for patient compliance. Azithromycin is a semi-synthetic derivative of erythromycin A. It is less potent than erythromycin against Gram-positive bacteria, but is more active against the Gram-negatives such as *H. influenzae*. Due to its long half-life it is normally administered once daily.

Telithromycin has activity against drug-resistant *S. pneumoniae*, regardless of the underlying resistance to other classes. It was withdrawn from general use in the United States in the late 1990s because of concerns about liver toxicity and its main use is for the treatment of resistant respiratory tract infections.

Lincosamides

The lincosamides are a small class of antibiotics with a structure unlike that of any of the other classes.

Route of administration: Parenteral administration can cause elevation of transaminases and serum alkaline phosphatase and may be complicated

---

Remember...

- *Aminoglycosides:* Used for treatment of serious infections. They are nephrotoxic and ototoxic and require routine monitoring
- *Tetracyclines and glycylcyclines:* Used predominantly for atypical coverage. Should not be given with milk as this reduces absorption
- *Macrolides and ketolides:* Used for atypical infections and often in penicillin-allergic patients. Interact with statins, causing myopathy and so should not be given concomittantly
- *Lincosamides:* Clindamycin is a high-risk antibiotic for *C. difficile* infection and its use within a hospital should be only in consultation with the microbiology or infectious diseases team

---

by thrombophlebitis. Rashes are an additional adverse reaction, and occur in approximately 10% of patients.

Clinical indications: Clinical use includes skin and soft tissue infections and osteomyelitis. It is a known high-risk antibiotic for *C. difficile* infection and should be used with great caution in elderly patients and those with predisposing factors to developing *C. difficile* infection (Dubberke et al 2008, Gerding et al 2008, Monaghan et al 2008). A risk–benefit analysis needs to be carried out before it is used in these patients.

Spectrum of use: Clindamycin has excellent bone penetration and has Gram-positive activity, including against MRSA and streptococci, but is not active against enterococci. Aerobic Gram-negative rods are uniformly resistant.

Other antibacterial agents

Quinupristin/dalfopristin

This is a combination of semi-synthetic streptogramin antibiotics (30:70).

Issues of administration: It is available only as an injection and needs to be administered via a central line (unless the first dose needs to be given as an emergency).

Clinical indications: Quinupristin/dalfopristin is used for the treatment of Gram-positive infections (includes methicillin-sensitive *Staphylococcus aureus*, MRSA, *S. pyogenes* and vancomycin-resistant *Enterococcus faecium;* it is *not* active against *E. faecalis*), which have not responded to previous antibacterial therapy, such as skin and soft tissue infections and hospital-acquired pneumonia.

Adverse effects include inflammation, pain, oedema, thrombophlebitis and injection site reactions when given via peripheral administration. It should not be administered if the plasma bilirubin concentration is more than three times the upper limit of the accepted reference range (Aksoy and Unal 2008, Barton and MacGowan 2009, Royal Pharmaceutical Society 2010).

Oxazolidinones

Oxazolidinones are unrelated to any other class of antibiotics (Finch et al 2003). They inhibit protein synthesis and are bacteriostatic against most bacteria. Linezolid is the most important member of the class.

Issues of administration: Oral and intravenous preparations are available. The oral tablets/suspension have 100% bioavailability (indicating that blood levels are equivalent if given via either route). Linezolid is given twice daily.

Clinical indications: Uses include complicated skin and soft tissue infections, osteomyelitis and ventilator-associated pneumonia (including MRSA pneumonia).

Gastrointestinal side-effects may occur, as well as other more serious side-effects such as optic neuropathy and blood disorders. This antibacterial agent is known to interact with monoamine oxidase inhibitors (MAOIs) and should not be given in conjunction with them (Aksoy and Unal 2008, Barton and MacGowan 2009, Royal Pharmaceutical Society 2010).

Spectrum of use: Linezolid has potent activity against Gram-positive organisms including MRSA and glycopeptide-resistant enterococci. Despite the relatively recent introduction of this compound, resistance has already been reported.

Daptomycin

Daptomycin is a cyclic lipopeptide antibiotic derived from *Streptomyces roseosporus*. The exact mechanism of action remains unknown.

Issues of administration: It is poorly absorbed orally and is only available as an IV preparation. It can be given once daily (Royal Pharmaceutical Society 2010).

Clinical indications: Daptomycin is indicated for the treatment of complicated skin and soft tissue infections (cSSSI), right-sided endocarditis (RIE) due to *S. aureus,* and *S. aureus* bacteraemia when associated with RIE or cSSSI.

It is extensively protein bound (90–95%) and is eliminated by the kidneys with a half-life of approximately 8 hours but rising to 30 hours in patients with renal impairment. Although generally well tolerated, various serious

---

Remember...

There are a number of antibacterials that can be used for the treatment of serious Gram-positive infections, especially if glycopeptides cannot be used. These include:

- *Quinupristin/dalfopristin:* Must be given via a central line and needs monitoring for potential side-effects, e.g. caution in hepatic dysfunction
- *Linezolid:* The oral preparations are 100% bioavailable. Serious side-effects include optic neuropathy and blood disorders
- *Daptomycin:* Only available as an intravenous preparation and given once daily. Side effects include muscle effects which could rarely produce rhabdomyolysis

adverse reactions have been reported, including muscle toxicity and elevated creatinine phosphokinase (Barton and MacGowan 2009). The latter should be routinely monitored prior to daptomycin therapy as well as during ongoing treatment. Daptomycin should not be administered concomitantly with HMG-CoA reductase inhibitors (i.e. statins). It is not licensed for the treatment of pneumonia. Clinical use is mostly in the treatment of complicated skin and soft-tissue infections. Daptomycin is a valuable agent, especially in cases where patients have renal dysfunction and cannot be given nephrotoxic antibacterial agents, e.g. vancomycin.

Spectrum of use: The spectrum of activity closely overlaps with that of the glycopeptides. It is highly active against MRSA and penicillin-resistant *Streptococcus pneumoniae* and is also active against some glycopeptide-resistant enterococci strains.

Rifampicin

Rifampicin is derived from rifamycin. Rifamycin is a natural antibiotic, first isolated from *Amycolatopsis mediterranei*.

Issues of administration: It is usually administered orally but intravenous preparations are available.

Clinical indications: Rifampicin is used for the treatment of tuberculosis, as well as other mycobacterial infections. It is also commonly used, in conjunction with other antibacterials, in the treatment of Gram-positive infections, e.g. staphylococci, due to its syngergistic effect.

Rifampicin is known to colour body secretions orange/red and patients (as well as healthcare professionals) must be aware of this. Side-effects include gastrointestinal effects and hepatotoxicity. Patients who are rifampicin-naïve should have a liver-function test taken prior to therapy. This drug is a potent inducer of the P-450 cytochrome system. It interacts with a large number of drugs and so concurrent medications must be checked for interactions prior to initiating therapy (Royal Pharmaceutical Society 2010).

Spectrum of use: Resistance develops rapidly and should be carefully monitored. Use as a single agent is strongly discouraged, but may be indicated as prophylaxis for secondary cases of *Haemophilus influenzae* Type b (Hib) or pneumococcal meningitis.

Fusidic acid

Fusidic acid and its salts, e.g. sodium fusidate, are narrow-spectrum antibacterial agents.

Issues of administration: It is available both as oral and intravenous preparations.

Clinical indications: Sodium fusidate has excellent bone penetration and is used for the treatment of staphylococcal osteomyelitis, as well as cellulitis, complicated skin and soft tissue infections and staphylococcal endocarditis.

Gastrointestinal side-effects may occur as well as more serious side-effects which include hepatotoxicity. If used in neonates, it may cause kernicterus.

Spectrum of use: It is regularly administered with rifampicin for the treatment of proven staphylococcal infections. It should not be used as a sole agent, due to the rapid development of resistance.

Metronidazole

Issues of administration: Preparations include oral, parenteral, topical and rectal with a high bioavailability achieved with all formulations.

Clinical indications: Indications include most anaerobic infections and some protozoal diseases such as *Gardnerella vaginalis*, dental infections, e.g. Vincent's angina, *Giardia lamblia* and *Entamoeba histolytica*, causative agents of Travellers' diarrhoea. Resistance to this agent has been described but is uncommon. It is used as a first-line treatment for *C. difficile* infection.

Side-effects include gastrointestinal effects, metallic taste, hepatotoxicity and peripheral neuropathy. The adverse effects of metronidazole are dose-related. Convulsive seizures and peripheral neuropathy have been reported as well as gastrointestinal disturbance. Metronidazole may produce a disulfiram-like effect if taken with alcohol.

Spectrum of use: Metronidazole has important Gram-negative and Gram-positive anaerobic activity. It is a potent inhibitor of obligate anaerobic bacteria and protozoa.

Co-trimoxazole

Co-trimoxazole (composed of sulphamethoxazole and trimethoprim) is a sulphonamide.

Issues of administration: Co-trimoxazole can be administred both orally and intravenously.

Clinical indications: Co-trimoxazole is now mostly reserved for the treatment of *Pneumocystis jirovecii*, toxoplasmosis and nocardiosis. It may be used for MRSA eradication, if sensitive, under supervision from the microbiology/infectious diseases team. Trimethoprim is a narrow spectrum agent which is commonly used for urinary tract infections but since resistance is prevalent, its use should only follow antibiotic susceptibility testing.

Co-trimoxazole may produce gastrointestinal side-effects, blood disorders, and Stevens-Johnson's syndrome, and needs adequate hydration to avoid crystalluria.

Spectrum of use: Since trimethoprim is a dihydrofolate reductase inhibitor, it (and co-trimoxazole) should not be used in conjunction with folate antagonists, such as methotrexate.

Stop, check, ask...

- Do you know where the following information can be found?
  - Antibiotic prescribing policy
  - Antibiotic guidelines
  - Information on the side-effects of antibiotics
- Who can you ask about the above if you cannot find the answer/information in your place of work?
- What are the clinical signs of a patient having an adverse effect to an antibacterial agent?
- If this happens on your ward, what would you do?

Medical device infections and treatment

As discussed in previous chapters, the term 'medical devices' is used to describe invasive appliances that are essentially foreign bodies. Examples of medical devices include: intravascular catheters, e.g. cerebrospinal fluid shunts; central venous and peripheral venous catheters; epidural and urinary catheters; prosthetic valves and joints; and continuous ambulatory peritoneal dialysis (CAPD) catheters.

The most common organisms that infect medical devices, especially in immunocompromised patients and where there is skin contact, are coagulase-negative staphylococci (biofilm producers) and *S. aureus* (including MRSA). Others, such as coliforms and *P. aeruginosa* are associated with infections in urinary catheters and endotracheal tubes. If infection develops, where possible, these devices should be removed. Empiric therapy should take into account target organisms, type of device and patient-specific factors (Elliott et al 2007).

Antibacterial prophylaxis

In order to prevent infections in specific exceptional circumstances, antibacterial prophylaxis may be required. Antibacterial prophylaxis may be indicated in certain serious conditions, or if patients are considered to be at high risk for developing post-operative infections (e.g. when undergoing abdominal surgery or before total knee/hip replacement surgery) which could potentially result in considerable morbidity and also mortality, if antibiotic prophylaxis is not given. Other examples would be in patients who have undergone elective or unplanned splenectomies, as these patients need to have life-long penicillin prophylaxis, in addition to vaccinations, in order to prevent a fatal pneumonia.

In addition, antibiotic prophylaxis would be needed for the prevention of bacterial meningitis in a close contact, prevention of gas-gangrene in a high risk patient or a secondary case of rheumatic fever (Royal Pharmaceutical Society 2010).

For surgical prophylaxis, one dose of antibiotic(s) is generally advised and it must be ensured that adequate levels of the antibiotic are present at the target site. It is recommended that antibiotic injections are administered 30–60 minutes prior to induction (Department of Health 2007, Cooke and Holmes 2007), except if rectal metronidazole is used. The latter necessitates 2 hours to elapse in order to achieve adequate levels (Munckhof 2005). Surgical operations which require routine antibiotic prophylaxis include: gastrointestinal, orthopaedic, urological, obstetric and gynaecological as well as vascular surgery. Local hospitals and clinics should have in-house, evidence-based guidelines, which take into account local epidemiological patterns. Until recently, parenteral cephalosporins were routinely used as surgical prophylaxis (together with metronidazole, where anaerobic infections may occur), however this is largely changing, due to their potential of inducing toxigenic *C. difficile* infection.

Key points

- If a client/patient has a medical device in place, check for signs of infection and report this immediately
- Be aware a patient may require antibacterial prophylaxis prior to a surgical procedure

---

Resistant mechanisms in bacteria

Although in the first part of this chapter, an overview of antibacterial agents currently in use were discussed, antibacterial resistance is a global and increasing phenomenon, affecting all the available classes of antibiotics currently in clinical use.

Infections such as MRSA, glycopeptide-resistant enterococci, drug-resistant *Streptococcus pneumoniae* (DRSP), ESBL-producing, as well as multi-drug-resistant Gram-negative bacteria (which includes enzymes such as SHV, VIM, AmpC and CTX-M) are referred to as healthcare-associated infections (HCAIs). These are monitored locally as well as internationally in most parts of the developed world.

Bacteria may become resistant to antibacterial agents using one or more of the following strategies (Alcamo 2001, Elliott et al 2007, Murray et al 2007, Greenwood et al 2008, McGavock 2008). *Figure 11.1* provides a pictorial illustration of these techniques:

1. Inactivation of antibacterial: For example, β-lactamases destroy the β-lactam ring in β-lactam antibiotics and, hence, the agent is rendered ineffective before penetrating the bacterial cell.
2. Target site modification: This can be achieved if there is a conformation change in the site of the action of the antibacterial, e.g. altered penicillin-binding proteins, as occurs in MRSA and penicillin-resistant pneumococci.
3. Efflux pumps: Some organisms, e.g. *Pseudomonas aeruginosa* pump out the antibiotic molecules on entry, preventing any adverse reaction on the bacterial cell, e.g. in quinolones.
4. Metabolic bypass: This occurs in sulphonamides and trimethoprim, where bacteria use essential elements from alternative sources, rather than synthesising their own, thereby bypassing the target enzyme for the antibiotic to act.
5. Target site protection: This occurs predominantly in ribosomes, where a conformational change would prevent the antibacterial from 'recognising' its target but would not have any deleterious effects on the bacterial cell.
6. Prevention of entry into bacterial cell: Uncommon and occurs in tetrayclines and aminoglycosides.

Other antimicrobials

In addition to antibacterials, other agents are commonly employed to treat infections.

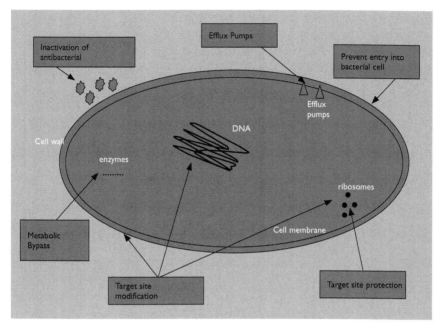

Figure 11.1: Bacterial resistance mechanisms.

Antifungals

Antifungal agents are used to combat fungal infections. Common preparations include:

- Polyene antifungals, e.g. amphotericin, used for the treatment of systemic fungal infections. These are given parenterally and are also available as lozenges. Amphotericin has a number of side-effects such as electrolyte disturbances, nephrotoxicity and hepatoxicity.
- Nystatin is another polyene that is available as a suspension and is used for the treatment of oesophageal and intestinal candidiasis.
- Triazole antifungals include fluconazole and voriconazole. These agents are used to treat fungal infections, typically *Candida* spp. and *Aspergillus* spp. Fluconazole is not active against *Aspergillus* spp. These drugs interact with numerous other drugs and care must be taken to ensure that there are no interacting medications before initiating therapy. An important interaction is that with statins. If a triazole is given concurrently with a statin, this may result in myopathy.

- The imidazoles, e.g. clotrimazole, econazole and miconazole, are used for the topical treatment of *Candida* and dermatophyte infections.
- Echinocandins, e.g. caspofungin, are used for the treatment of systemic fungal infections and these drugs have fewer interactions than the triazoles.

Antivirals

Antiviral agents are used to treat viral infections. The drug aciclovir is the drug of choice for herpes virus infections. It is available topically, orally and intravenously. Antivirals used for the prophylaxis and treatment of influenza are oseltamivir (available orally) and zanamavir (inhaler). A number of antiviral agents are used for the treatment of human immunodeficiency virus (HIV), a retrovirus, and these act by inhibiting the activity of HIV. Anti-retrovirals are used as a combination, in order to prevent the emergence of resistance.

In addition to antiviral and antifungal agents, antiparasitic agents are used for parasitic infections. An important example is malaria; a well-known antimalarial drug is quinine.

Antimicrobial stewardship

Antimicrobial management teams (AMT) are a key tool to help control the dissemination and emergence of new resistant microorganisms, including fungi, viruses, and parasites, as well as bacteria. Infection control and antimicrobial management or stewardship should be combined as a multi-faceted approach (see *Figure 11.2*). The following includes a set of basic principles that should be rigorously adopted by all clinicians and independent prescribers when considering antimicrobial therapy for patients.

Top tips for safe and rational antimicrobial prescribing

Clinical indication of antimicrobials
- Antimicrobials are indicated only if the patient exhibits clinical signs and/or symptoms of infection or sepsis (Cooke and Holmes 2007, Department of Health and Health Protection Agency 2009, RCP 2009), e.g. temperature higher than 38°C or lower than 36°C, increasing (or low for certain systemic infections, e.g. CA-MRSA) white cell count, increasing inflammatory markers, e.g. high C-reactive protein, erythrocyte sedimentation rate or biomarkers, e.g. high pro-calcitonin specifically denotes bacterial infection.

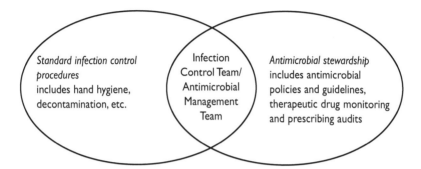

Figure 11.2. An effective basic strategy that should be adopted by infection control and antimicrobial management teams.

Antimicrobial agent selection

- Identify any allergies to antimicrobials and document them; if unclear, ask patient directly.
- Adhere to the local, evidence-based antimicrobial guidelines (Department of Health 2007, RCP 2009).
- Use culture and sensitivity results, if available and if not, take relevant specimens prior to starting antimicrobial therapy, unless infection is life-threatening, e.g. meningitis. Refer to results when available and change prescription accordingly (Department of Health 2003, 2007, Cooke and Holmes 2007, Dellit et al 2007, Royal College of Physicians 2009).
- Use of broad-spectrum agents should be avoided wherever possible (e.g. cephalosporins, fluoroquinolones and co-amoxiclav) and narrow-spectrum agents encouraged (Department of Health 2003, 2007, Dellit et al 2007).
- If in doubt, seek immediate advice from the microbiologist and/or infectious diseases physician prior to prescribing.

Appropriate route and duration

- Oral antimicrobials should be prescribed as first choice, unless the infection is life-threatening or severe (e.g. neutropenic sepsis, endocarditis, meningitis, etc). If specific patient factors prevent this (e.g. inability to swallow) or if the preferred agent can only be given parenterally (e.g. tigecycline, daptomycin, etc.) then they should be administered intravenously, intramuscularly or rectally.
- Oral antimicrobials should be prescribed for a maximum of five days and re-prescribed (and re-written on the medication chart) if needed for longer

(Department of Health 2007).

- Each antimicrobial agent given parenterally should be prescribed for a maximum of 48 hours and if needed for a longer period, this should be recorded on the medication chart.

Daily review of antimicrobials

- Antimicrobial therapy should be reviewed on a daily basis by the clinical team during the ward round.
- Documentation supporting daily review should be clearly evident from the patient's medical notes.

Surgical prophylaxis

- One dose is indicated pre-operatively (unless otherwise proven for specific conditions by evidence-based guidelines) (Cooke and Holmes 2007, Department of Health 2007).
- A second dose may be needed if the procedure lasts for four or more hours, or if there is excessive blood loss (Department of Health 2007). Microbiological advice should always be sought, if unsure.

Checklist to ensure good antimicrobial stewardship

☐ Establish a local antimicrobial management team with regular documented meetings

☐ Local evidence-based antimicrobial guidelines for prophylaxis and treatment of infections

☐ Antimicrobial formulary

☐ IV to oral switch policy or automatic IV stop dates

☐ Procedure in place for the supply of restricted antimicrobials

☐ Therapeutic drug monitoring service, with appropriate guidance

☐ Ongoing clinical education on antimicrobial prescribing

☐ Antimicrobial prescribing audit programme, including retrospective and prospective audits and dissemination of results to clinical staff

Adapted from: MacDougall et al 2005, Dellit et al 2007, Department of Health 2007

Summary

This chapter looked at a wide range of antibacterial agents used to combat infections. The historical perspective and developments over the last century were outlined. The classification of various antibacterial agents as well as their key properties, including side-effect profile and interactions were discussed. An overview of the challenges of resistance mechanisms commonly found in bacteria that render certain antibacterials ineffective, thus necessitating the use of stronger agents with potentially serious side-effects, was presented. This calls for judicious use of all antimicrobial agents and multidisciplinary teamworking alongside infection control and antimicrobial management teams in order to promote antimicrobial stewardship, thereby providing our patients with optimal care.

In the final chapter we will look at the roles and responsibilites of staff involved not only in the prescribing and managment of antimicrobial agents, but also in other aspects of the prevention and control of infections within a healthcare organisation.

Acknowledgements

The editorial support of Ms Annie M Jones (MSC Ltd) is acknowledged in the preparation of this chapter.

References

Aksoy DY, Unal S (2008) New antimicrobial agents for the treatment of Gram-positive bacterial infections. *Clinical Microbiology and Infection* **14**: 411–20

Alcamo IE (ed) (2001) *Fundamentals of microbiology* (6th edn). Jones and Bartlett Publishers, Canada

Barton E, MacGowan A (2009) Future treatment options for Gram-positive infections – looking ahead. *Clinical Microbiology and Infection* **15**(Suppl 6): 17–25

Cooke FJ, Holmes AH (2007) The missing care bundle; antibiotic prescribing in hospitals. *International Journal of Antimicrobial Agents* **30**: 25–9

Dancer S (2008) The effect of antibiotics on methicillin-resistant *Staphylococcus aureus*. *Journal of Antimicrobial Chemotherapy* **61**: 246–53

Dellit TH, Owens RC, McGowan JE et al (2007) Infectious Diseases Society of America and the Society for Healthcare Epidemiology of America Guidelines for Developing an Institutional Program to Enhance Antimicrobial Stewardship. *Clinical Infectious*

Diseases **44**: 159–77

Department of Health (2003) *Winning Ways: Working together to reduce healthcare associated infection in England*. Department of Health, London

Department of Health (2007) *Saving Lives: Reducing infection, delivering clean and safe care*. Department of Health, London

Department of Health (2009) *The Health and Social Care Act 2008. Code of practice for the health and adult social care on the prevention and control of health care associated infections and related guidance*. Department of Health, London

Department of Health and Health Protection Agency (2009) *Clostridium difficile infection: How to deal with the problem*. Department of Health, London

Dubberke ER, Gerding DN, Classen D, et al (2008) Strategies to prevent *Clostridium difficile* infections in acute care hospitals. *Infection Control and Hospital Epidemiology* **29**: S81–92

Elliott T, Worthington T, Osman H, Gill M (2007) *Lecture Notes: Medical Microbiology and Infection* (4th edn). Blackwell Publishing, Oxford

Finch RG, Greenwood D, Norrby SR, Whitley RJ (eds) (2003) *Antibiotic and chemotherapy: Anti-infective agents and their use in therapy* (8th edn). Churchill Livingstone, New York

Frankland P, Frankland GC (1901) *Pasteur*. Cassell, London

Gerding DN, Muto CA, Owens RC (2008) Measures to control and prevent *Clostridium difficile* infection. *Clinical Infectious Diseases* 46: S43–9

Greenwood D, Finch R, Davey P, Wilcox M (2008) *Antimicrobial chemotherapy* (5th edn). Oxford University Press, Oxford

Hauser AR (2007) *Antibiotic basics for clinicians: Choosing the right antibacterial agent*. Lippincott Williams & Wilkins, Baltimore MD

Infectious Diseases Society of America (2010) The 10 X '20 Initiative: Pursuing a global commitment to develop 10 new antibacterial drugs by 2020. *Clinical Infectious Diseases* **50**: 1081–3

Kisgen J, Whitney D (2008) Ceftobiprole, a broad-spectrum cephalosporin with activity against MRSA. *Pharmacy and Therapeutics* **33**(11): 631–41

Liebowitz LD, Blunt MC (2008) Modification in prescribing practices for third generation cephalosporins and ciprofloxacin is associated with a reduction in methicillin-resistant *Staphylococcus aureus* bacteraemia rate. *Journal of Hospital infection* **69**: 328–36

MacDougall C, Polk RE (2005) Antimicrobial stewardship programs in healthcare systems. *Clinical Microbiology Reviews* **18**(4): 638–56

Mandell GL, Bennett JE, Dolin R (eds) (2009) *Mandell, Douglas and Bennett's principles and practice of infectious diseases* (7th edn). Churchill Livingstone, New York

McGavock H (2008) *How drugs work. Basic pharmacology for healthcare professionals* (2nd edn). Radcliffe Publishing, Oxford

Monaghan T, Boswell T, Mahida YR (2008) Recent advances in *Clostridium difficile*-associated disease. *Gut* **57**(6): 850–60

Munckhof W (2005) Antibiotics for surgical prophylaxis. *Australian Prescriber* **28**(2): 38–40

Murray PR, Baron EJ, Jorgensen JH, Landry ML, Pfaller M (eds) (2007) *Manual of clinical microbiology* (9th edn) Vol 1. American Society for Microbiology Press, Washington DC

Nicolau DP, Freeman CD, Belliveau PP, et al (1995) Experience with a once-daily aminoglycoside program administered to 2,184 adult patients. *Antimicrobial Agents and Chemotherapy* **39**(3): 650–5

Owens JC, Donskey CJ, Gaynes RP, et al (2008) Antimicrobial-associated risk factors for *Clostridium difficile* infection. *Clinical Infectious Diseases* **46**: S19–31

Paterson DL (2004) 'Collateral damage' from cephalosporin or quinolone antibiotic therapy. *Clinical Infectious Diseases* **38**(Suppl 4): S341–5

Royal College of Physicians Healthcare Associated Infection Working Group (2009) *Short guidelines for optimal hospital antimicrobial prescribing*. Available from: http:www.rcplondon.ac.uk [Accessed 11 December 2009].

Royal Pharmaceutical Society (2010) *British National Formulary (BNF 60)*. British Medical Association and Royal Pharmacuetical Society of Great Britain, London

Tacconelli E, De Angelis, Cataldo MA, et al (2008) Does antibiotic exposure increase the risk of methicillin-resistant *Staphylococcus aureus* (MRSA) isolation? A systematic review and meta-analysis. *Journal of Antimicrobial Chemotherapy* **61**(1): 26–38

Wilcox MH, Mooney L, Bendall R, et al (2008) A case-control study of community-associated *Clostridium difficile* infection. *Journal of Antimicrobial Chemotherapy* **62**: 388–90

World Health Organization (2009) *World Health Statistics*. Available from: http://www.who.int/whosis/whostat/EN_WHS09_Full.pdf. [Accessed 5 April 2010]

CHAPTER 12

Infection prevention and control: Roles and responsibilities

Vinice Thomas

Purpose

The purpose of this chapter is to provide an outline of some of the key roles and responsibilities of staff working within health and social care to prevent and control infections.

Learning outcomes

By the end of this chapter, you will have learned:

- The core responsibilities of staff to prevent infections.
- The role of the board in achieving reductions in healthcare-associated infections.
- The key roles of the infection prevention and control team.
- How to ensure you fulfil your role as a worker within a care setting in order to prevent infection and cross-infection.

Introduction

Previous chapters looked at some of the components of care that are vital to infection prevention and control. It is clear that the infection prevention and control agenda is so vast that it is impossible to be fulfilled by any one person or group of staff (National Audit Office 2009). Commitment of the whole healthcare system is required to achieve a reduction in healthcare-associated infections (HCAIs), to realise the aim of improving the quality of care provided, and to ensure patients' safety (Department of Health 2008a).

Throughout all stages of the patient's health and social care journey, the complexity of care and the number of healthcare workers likely to contribute to recovery increase exposure to the risks of HCAIs. As a result, all levels of staff need to work together with the infection prevention and control team to tackle

HCAIs (Department of Health 2008b). A sustainable reduction in HCAIs is achievable if there is joined up working from board level to the frontline of care, and from community settings to the heart of a busy acute healthcare organisation. There is a real need for all parties to clearly understand and fulfil their individual roles and responsibilities, and to work in partnership across professional and healthcare boundaries.

General roles and responsibilities

As outlined in *Figure 12.1*, infection control is everyone's business; this includes an array of staff with different roles and responsibilities (Department of Health 2008b). It is commonplace to find roles that are interlinked and therefore

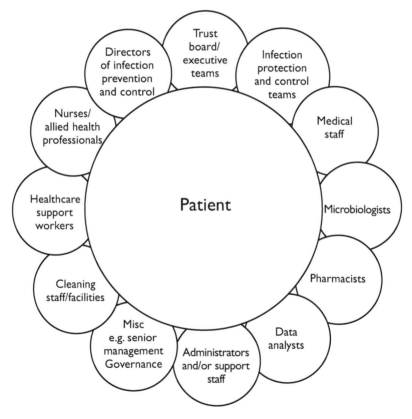

Figure 12.1. Key roles supporting the infection prevention and control agenda.

dependant on one another to function effectively, such as the junior doctors, registered nurses, and healthcare support workers. Collaborative working and an understanding of each unique role are integral to effective teamwork and cohesive seamless care to patients. However, this requires an organisational culture of 'zero tolerance' towards poor performance and standards, incidents of HCAIs, and dysfunctional teams.

To inform staff of what is expected of them, it is important that this is clearly outlined within all job descriptions, is a feature when setting individual objectives, and is in personal development plans and appraisals. There is commonality in some aspects of the roles and responsibilities. For instance all staff are responsible for undertaking the relevant training sessions and updates as part of their continuous professional development.

The organisation's policies and guidelines highlight the expected performance/ procedures to be applied by staff, and therefore it is vital staff familiarise themselves with these. These include infection control-related policies, cleaning and decontamination procedures, how to report risks, etc. Infection risks are significantly reduced when staff consistently apply best practice, as outlined in procedures and policies, thus minimising any variation in the standard of care.

In the event of a patient incident/accident, staff are responsible for contributing to and cooperating with any investigations as deemed appropriate by the investigating officer. Within the context of infection prevention and control, this may mean participating in root cause analysis investigations into a methicillin-resistant *Staphylococcus aureus* (MRSA) bacteraemia cases or *Clostridium difficile* outbreaks.

Summary of general roles and responsibilities

- Value the contribution of other team members
- Attend infection control updates/training
- Familiarise yourself with policies and procedures and ensure these are applied consistently
- Fulfil the infection prevention and control role as outlined within job descriptions
- Achieve the infection prevention and control objectives outlined within personal development plans
- Co-operate with clinical investigations as deemed appropriate

---

Trust board

The trust board (or equivalent) is in a prime position to steer and lead the organisation to become an exemplary provider of quality care. More recently boards are operating within a climate where they are subject to close scrutiny by regulators, media and patient groups and face the challenge of managing financial constraints and competing priorities whilst having to ensure safety remains at the forefront of their agenda.

The board has a responsibility to set the strategic direction of the organisation and communicate a clear vision and purpose to staff; one that will unite staff groups around common goals and values. A clear communication strategy that cascades the value and vision to staff is invaluable to obtain staff commitment and engagement. Furthermore, a culture must be created which is open, positive and transparent, where staff feel valued and able to raise concerns. An adverse culture will have an adverse effect on staff morale and on the confidence of staff to express genuine safety issues, as was the case in a recent HCAI-related incident (Health Care Commission 2009). Therefore, board members must be visible to staff and approachable (Department of Health 2008b).

All staff need to be aware of their responsibilities within the legal requirements of the Health and Social Care Act (2008), often referred to as the Hygiene Code, and need robust processes and systems within which to operate to fulfil their duties. The board needs to ensure these processes and systems are in place and be assured that they are working effectively and efficiently. Board assurance relies on timely and credible data/information that demonstrate how well the board is performing against its targets and corporate objectives. This is one of the key responsibilities of the chief executive officer (CEO), i.e. assuring the board of the quality of the service and that corporate and clinical governance systems are in place. However, the CEO must hold the other directors to account for the HCAI performance within their departments, e.g. achieving local targets which have been disseminated to the clinical areas and are the prime responsibility of clinical leaders such as matrons/ward managers.

The use of dashboards containing key performance indicators around HCAIs is one way of monitoring performance. These performance indicators can include outcomes on infection rates, audit results for hand hygiene, and root cause analysis, and can be presented in a 'user-friendly' format, such as a series of graphs. Many healthcare organisations within the UK use these to good effect.

It is widely recognised that staff closest to patients have the biggest impact on their care, experience and satisfaction. The board is responsible for ensuring adequate resource and support is made available to equip staff to fulfil their roles, e.g. staffing levels, training budgets (Health and Social Care Act 2008).

As depicted in *Figure 12.2*, the board is influential in equipping staff and setting the stage for best practice and a positive learning culture (Health Care Commission 2009). This has an impact on staff at all levels (as shown in *Figure 12.2*). The staff are influential in directly impacting the experience of patients and this increases to some extent the closer the staff member is to frontline care. This highlights the interdependency of the board and frontline staff, and the importance of board-to-ward engagement.

Visible and strong leadership is required at every level of the organisation in order to achieve and sustain improvement in patient care and a reduction in HCAIs.

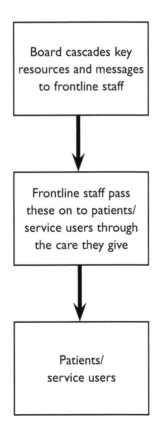

Figure 12.2. A team approach to impact patient care.

One of the board's key roles is to provide and model quality leadership and foster it at all levels of the organisation. One way this has been achieved successfully is by board members visiting clinical areas and meeting with staff and patients. This has provided opportunities for board members to see at first hand the good work and challenges occurring within the clinical area.

Table 12.1 outlines specific roles held by members of the board.

Table 12.1. Executive board: Role titles and responsibilities	
Title	*Key responsibilities/duties*
Director of infection prevention and control	• Oversees the infection prevention and control agenda and related policies • Ensures good antibiotic stewardship and challenges inappropriate prescribing practices • Reports directly to the board on HCAI issues and performance (Department of Health 2004a) • Presents annual infection prevention and control report (Department of Health 2008c)
Nurse and medical directors	• Lead on HCAI-related improvement plans and engage members of the workforce • Take the lead on HCAI-related serious untoward incidents • Oversee root cause analysis and ensure dissemination of learning across the organisation • Obtain HCAI-related data that contribute to the key performance indicators
Human resources director	• Ensures HCAI is within each job description • Ensures monitoring and delivery of HCAI-related training
Financial director	• Quantifies the financial savings from HCAI improvement and reports to the board • Monitors and reports financial impact of antibiotic use and screening as well as other HCAI initiatives
Non-executive directors	• Scrutinise and challenge HCAI performance data • Champion HCAI agenda to staff and external partners
	Adapted from Department of Health (2008c)

Summary of responsibilities of trust boards

- Set clear vision and strategic direction
- Communicate values and vision to staff
- Demonstrate strong and visible leadership
- Ensure efficient resource allocation and investments
- Monitor the performance of the trust
- Ensure clear communication strategy for liaising with the general public and the media on HCAI performance

---

Infection prevention and control team

The infection prevention and control team consists of infection control nurses (registered nurses who have undertaken specialist training in infection control), trainee infection control nurses, infection control doctor/microbiologist and the director of infection prevent and control mentioned in the previous section. It is important to note that some care settings do not employ an infection control doctor, so it is important that staff have access to one through some other contractual arrangements, or a consultant in health protection (Hygiene Code 2008).

Another role that is important for the organisation is the decontamination lead. This is usually fulfilled as part of an existing infection prevention and control role, and must be included when establishing infection prevention and control teams. Working closely with the infection prevention and control team, and in some organisations being an integral part of the team, are the antimicrobial pharmacist and data analyst.

The team plays a central role in the development of the HCAI programme of work which ensures the organisation complies with the Hygiene Code (Health and Social Care Act 2008). Through an annual work plan, the team delivers the programme as well as a corporate training schedule and audit timetable. The team leads in the review of infection prevention and control-related policies, ensuring these are in line with national guidelines and best practice.

The team provides leadership and expertise to the wider healthcare organisation (Department of Health 2008b); this includes providing advice on the use of HCAI-related tools and procedures, such as the Department of Health (2005) Saving Lives tool, and root cause analysis investigations.

As infection control is 'everyone's business' (Health Care Commission 2007),

229

Table 12.2. Key roles of the infection prevention and control team

Title	Summary of some key responsibilities/duties
Infection control nurse	• Provides advice and leadership across the organisation • Supports data collection of HCAI indicators • Delivers HCAI programme with the support of the clinical team • Helps with surveillance of infections
Microbiologist	• Advises on the antimicrobial agents best suited for the microorganisms • Plays a key role in the analysis of microorganisms • Has an advisory role to the wider organisation
Antimicrobial pharmacist	• Promotes good prescribing practices (Department of Health 2008a) • Supports the pharmacist by providing advice and help with audits
Data analyst	• Supports with the analysis and presentation of HCAI data • Advises and supports with the development of HCAI dashboards
	Adapted from Department of Health (2008c)

the infection prevention and control team facilitates infection control activities within clinical areas, such as the commencement of MRSA protocol, or screening. A facilitative role is vital as the team is not directly involved with the day-to-day clinical duties or patient care to the same degree as ward clinical staff. The team works with the clinical teams and departments to deliver the HCAI programme of work, and gather the necessary data/information related to HCAI systems, process and policies.

Table 12.2 outlines some of the key roles of the infection prevention and control team and related staff.

Clinical teams

Clinical teams are at the forefront of care and are key in preventing the spread of infections. As a result, it is vital they cooperate with the infection prevention and control team and participate in related activities such as training sessions, medical device updates, clinical audits, and root cause analysis investigations into serious infections, such as MRSA bacteraemia.

Audit

The clinical team will be expected to be involved with reviewing the standards of care given to the client and this is often through participating in clinical audits where the practice of staff is observed and compared with the policy/guidelines of the organisation. The results are recorded on a data collection tool, and are analysed to determine areas for improvement, and any necessary actions required. It is important that the lessons learned from the audit studies are shared with staff both within the original department and from other clinical areas. In some cases it has been considered beneficial for staff from other clinical areas to compare their results as well as share the learning. To ensure the audits are carried out using a robust and thorough technique, it is good practice for staff to undertake audits for other clinical areas and not their own as this has been found to reduce the likelihood of clinical staff altering their behaviour due to being observed by their own line manager.

Root cause analysis

In the event of the patient/service user acquiring an infection, i.e. bacteraemia, it is necessary to undertake an investigation to identify the cause of the infection and steps that may be taken to prevent a recurrence. The clinical team will need to participate in such an investigation, and contribute to fact finding and discussion of the likely causes of the infection. The findings of the root cause analysis will be disseminated to other departments in order to share the learning and apply the recommendations.

Surveillance

The infection prevention and control team needs to ensure that surveillance takes place within the clinical areas in line with national policies and local guidelines, that the results are followed up in a timely manner, and that appropriate actions are taken. Surveillance can highlight activities occurring within the clinical environment/organisation and identify trends and incidences. This is important in influencing practice and effective resource management, which are vital to reducing infections.

Table 12.3 outlines some of the key roles of the clinical staff.

Table 12.3. Key roles of clinical staff

Title	Summary of some key responsibilities/duties
Matron	• Ensures best practice is applied in relation to infection prevention and control in clinical areas • Works with the facilities team and cleaners to ensure provision of a clean environment • Improves clinical standards (Department of Health 2004b)
Ward manager/team leader	• Reports and shares HCAI data and information with staff, e.g. root cause analysis findings, hand hygiene data • Implements locally HCAI tools, e.g. audits, root cause analysis • Ensures staff are trained and follow best practice
Doctors	• Adhere to antibiotic prescribing policies • Ensure correct procedure and hygiene is maintained when inserting and examining medical devices
Nurses/healthcare support workers	• Ensure environment and equipment are cleaned according to local and national policies • Observe the correct procedure for caring for patients/clients with medical devices in situ • Participate in the relevant audits
Link nurses	• Reinforce best practice within the clinical areas • Support with infection prevention and control training and audits • Interface between ward and prevention and control team
	Adapted from Department of Health (2008c)

Facilities team

Cleaning within the healthcare environment can be generally separated into nursing or domestic/facilities cleaning. Medical devices and nursing equipment, such as nursing trolleys, will often be the responsibility of the nursing staff. Specialist medical devices that need sterilisation may be sent to a centralised sterilisation department, whereas the environment and certain furniture items, such as beds, will often be the responsibility of the domestic/facilities staff (this can vary according to local protocols). To achieve high standards of cleanliness, cleaners must undergo regular training, support and supervision. Their role is vital in reducing infection and cross-infection; therefore training updates must include best practice around choosing and using the correct cleaning solutions, use of cleaning equipment, and general safety advice.

The facilities team and ward team have to work closely together to minimise any items of equipment/furniture 'falling in the gap' between the staff groups. Therefore, a clear cleaning schedule and work programmes that identify roles and responsibilities of all parties is paramount. In addition, the teams need to participate in auditing the standard of cleanliness within the environment.

The role of the patient environment action team is important to provide independent assessment of the standards of cleanliness. All staff groups need to work in collaboration with patient environment action teams and implement any recommendations made.

Table 12.4 outlines some of the key roles of staff.

Patients/visitors

The organisation must have a clear communication strategy that outlines how it communicates with external stakeholders, such as patients, visitors, and the media. It can include information on how the organisation is performing in terms of reducing HCAIs, and success stories of staff innovations that have led to a reduction in infections.

Table 12.4. Key roles of facilities staff	
Title	*Summary of some key responsibilities/duties*
Head of facilities	• Ensures facilities comply with local and national standards, e.g. Hygiene Code 2008 • Oversees standards of cleanliness • Leads/participates in cleanliness audits
Domestic staff	• Work with the nursing staff to maintain a clutter-free and clean environment • Participate in cleaning audits and actions • Adhere to local cleaning protocols, policies and procedures
Adapted from Department of Health (2008c)	

Within healthcare there is a renewed emphasis on the patient–staff relationship where both parties are equal decision-makers in the patient's care. It is therefore beneficial for patients/visitors to work with health and social care staff to reduce infections by adhering to hand hygiene and other infection prevention and control practices (Department of Health 2008b). There has been a greater emphasis on this through the 'cleanyourhands' campaign (National Patient Safety Agency 2004), which has had a positive impact in many clinical areas.

In addition, the healthcare worker needs to ensure patients and visitors have access to information on infections, and are aware of other restrictions, such as barrier nursing, which may directly affect them. In some healthcare organisations in the UK, MRSA bacteraemia rates and hand hygiene audit results have been displayed so the general public can view the organisation's performance. This has been well received by patients who are able to use this information to assure themselves of the standards of hygiene within the trust.

Summary

This chapter has highlighted some of the key roles of staff working within executive boards, infection prevention and control teams, clinical teams and facilities teams. It is intended that the roles outlined will help to increase readers' awareness of the uniqueness of each staff group in contributing to the infection prevention and control agenda.

Preceding chapters have given overviews of the foundations of infection control, and it is hoped will have provided an incentive for further study and development in this stimulating and rewarding aspect of patient care.

References

Department of Health (2004a) *Competencies for director of infection prevention and control*. Department of Health, London

Department of Health (2004b) *A matron's charter: An action plan for cleaner hospitals*. Department of Health, London

Department of Health (2005) *Saving lives: Delivery programme to reduce HCAIs, including MRSA*. Department of Health, London

Department of Health (2008a) *Clean, safe care. Reducing infections and saving lives*. Department of Health, London

Department of Health (2008b) *Board to ward – how to embed a culture of HCAI preven-*

tion in acute trusts. Department of Health, London

Department of Health (2008c) *Reducing healthcare-associated infections: From trust board to ward*. Department of Health, London

Health Care Commission (2007) *Healthcare-associated infections: What else can the NHS do?* Health Care Commission, London

Health Care Commission (2009) *Investigation into Mid-Staffordshire NHS Foundation Trusts*. Health Care Commission, London

Health and Social Care Act (2008) *Code of Practice for health and adult social care on the prevention and control of infections and related guidance*. Department of Health, London

National Audit Office (2009) *Reducing healthcare-associated infections in hospitals in England*. National Audit Office, London

National Patient Safety Agency (2004) *Cleanyourhands campaign*. NPSA, London

Useful website

Patient Environment Action Team Inspections: www.npsa.nhs.uk/peat

Index

A

acid-fast bacilli 22
Acinetobacter spp. 21, 202
aerosol-generating procedures 121–123
AIDS 58
airborne transmission 31
alcohol hand gel 116
aminoglycosides
  administration 205
  clinical indications 205
  use 205
amoebic dysentery 24
amoxicillin 198
Amycolatopsis mediterranei 211
antibacterial
  agents
    mode of action 195–197
    timeline 194
  prophylaxis 214
antifungals 216
antimicrobials 215
  administration of 218
  clinical indications 217
  prescribing 217
antivirals 217
arsphenamine 194
artificial insemination 32
asepsis
  and invasive devices 158
aseptic technique 25, 158
  checklist 159
Aspergillus
  fumigates 23
  spp. 216

B

bacteraemia 20
bacteria 11–12
  resistant mechanisms in 215
  shape of 12
  spore-forming 14
  types of 13
Bacteroides fragilis 199
BCG 49, 54
bilharzia 35
biofilm 146, 161, 170, 172, 213
blood-borne virus 29, 55
  management of exposure to 125
body fluids
  management of 122
Bordetella pertussis 208
Borrelia burgdorferi 33, 206
Broad Street pump 10
burns 36

C

campylobacter 51
Candida spp. 216
carbapenems
  administration 202
  clinical indications 202
  use 202
carboxypenicillin 199
Care Quality Commission 72
  audit 85
  concerns about cleanliness 85

audit
  clinical 231
autoclave 105

catheter
  urinary 39
catheter-associated urinary tract
  infection (CAUTI) 170
catheters 38
cellulitis 28
cephalosporin 199–200
  clinical indications 200
  issues of administration 200
  susceptible bacteria 201
  use 200
Cephalosporium acremonium 200
chickenpox 49, 89
  see varicella-zoster virus
chilling
  of food 138
Chlamydia 35
  trachomatis 35, 207
cirrhosis 58, 59
cleaning 102
  deep 82
  definitions 73
  environmental 77
  for aesthetic reasons 74
  frequency of 80
  holistic approach 90
  key factors in 78
  key roles in 79
  manual 102
  methods 81
  monitoring and audit 83
  obstacles to 72
  periodic 82
  of equipment 86
  reasons for 74
  responsibility matrix 78
  risk categories 81
  schedules 80
  standard 77, 82
  steam 86

to prevent and control infection
  75–76
  training 83
cleanliness
  external regulator of 72
clinical
  staff
    key roles of 232
  teams 230
Clostridium
  difficile 1, 20, 76–77, 89, 114,
    116–117, 189, 200, 203, 204,
    209, 212, 214, 225
  perfringens 21, 135
  spp. 198
  tetani 21
co-amoxiclav 199
cockroaches 140
commensals 11
common vehicle spread 30
  blood and blood products 31
  case study 31
contact
  precautions 186
  transmission 29
Corynebacterium
  jeikeium 207
  spp. 205
co-trimoxazole
  administration 212
  clinical indications 212
  side-effects 213
  use 213
Creutzfeldt-Jakob disease (CJD) 98
  NICE recommendations 99
cross-contamination 136
  prevention of 137
Cryptosporidium spp. 24, 34
curtains 127
cystic fibrosis 30

D

daptomycin
  administration 210
  clinical indications 210
  side effects 210
  use 211
decontamination 73, 74
  cycle 101
  methods 100
  microbicidal activity of 106
  of instruments 98
deep cleaning 82
dental
  caries 35
  decontamination of instruments 108
  route of transmission 30
dermatitis 62, 63
devices
  intravenous access 163
diarrhoea
  infective 188
diphtheria 49
disinfection 73, 74, 81, 103
droplet transmission 30
ducts 88

E

ectoparasites 35
endocarditis 37
endophthalmitis 37
Entamoeba histolytica 24, 212
Enterobacteriaceae 202
Enterococcus
  faecalis 18, 201
  faecium 209
  spp. 207, 139
enterocolitis 20
EPIC Guidelines 114
Escherichia coli 11, 13, 19, 40, 51

estates department 87
eukaryotic cells 11
executive board
  roles and responsibilities 228
eye protection 121

F

face masks 121
facilities staff
  key roles of 233
  team 232–233
facultative anaerobes 13
faecal–oral route 34
  of transmission 30
Fleming, Alexander 194
flucloxacillin 198
fluoroquinolones
  administration 204
  clinical indications 204
  side effects 204
  use 205
Foley catheter 40,, 169
food
  cooking of 139
  hygiene 136
food-borne illness 29
fungi 14, 23
fusidic acid 211
  administration 212
  clinical indications 212
  side effects 212
  use 212
Fusobacterium spp. 198

G

Gardnerella vaginalis 212
gastroenteritis 51
Giardia 33, 34
  intestinalis 34

lamblia 212
gloves 120
glycopeptides
  administration 203
  clinical indications 203
  use 203
glycylcyclines
  administration 207
  clinical indications 207
  side effects 207
  use 207
gonorrhoea 35, 204
Gram-negative
  cocci 17–18
  bacteria 12
  rods 19
Gram stain 11

H

haemophilia 31
Haemophilus
  influenzae 202, 208
  spp. 208
hand hygiene 63, 114–115, 136, 159
  five moments of 64, 116
  technique 117
helminths 33, 34
hepatitis B virus 23, 49, 55, 58, 59,
  124–125
hepatitis C virus 23, 31, 55, 59, 60,
  124–125
herpes virus 58
Hickman lines 38
High Efficiency Particulate Air
  (HEPA) filters 89
High Impact Intervention Care bundle
  83
HIV 23, 29, 32, 55, 58, 124–125
  incubation and symptoms 58
  prevention 58

treatment 58
hospital-acquired infection 202
humidity 88
Hygiene Code 226

I

ice makers 140, 142
  best practice 143
immunisation 25, 48
impetigo 28
incineration 74
infection
  assessment of 183
  chain of 23, 24, 24–25
  control
    audit 84
    strategy for 218
  elements of transmission 29
  incubation periods 182
  of wounds 186
  policies and guidelines 187
  prevalence of 181–182
  prevention and control
    education 65–66
    key roles of 230
    roles and responsibilities 224
    team 229
  principles of treatment 183–184
  psychological effects of 4
  reservoir of 24
  route of entry 25
  route of transmission 25
  susceptible hosts 25
  vector-borne 33
infectious disease
  historical perspective 194
influenza 50, 53
  incubation and symptoms 53
  prevention 53
  treatment 53

inoculation injuries 56
intravenous
  access devices 163–169
  catheters 37, 163
  devices
    key points 169
    prevention of infection in 165
    types of infection 163
invasive devices
  documentation 161
  examples of 155
  functions of 156
  infection risks of 156
  management of 162
  preparation of the site 160
  prevention of infection in 157
isolation procedures 122–123

K

ketolides
  administration 207
  clinical indications 207
  use 207
Klebsiella pneumoniae 19, 139, 140,
    202

L

Lancefield groups 18
latex sensitivity 62
laundry
  categories of 126
Legionella 89, 136, 140, 146
legionnaires' disease 136, 146
  risk assessment 147
leukaemia 58
lincosamides
  administration 208
  clinical indications 208
  use 208

linen
  colour standards for 126
  management of 125–126
  rules for handling 127
Listeria spp. 198
Lyme disease 33

M

macrolides
  administration 207
  indications 207
  use 207
malaria 24, 33, 217
matron 78, 84
mattress audit 84
measles, mumps and rubella (MMR)
    48
medical devices
  infection of 213
Mellon, Mary 50
meningitis 19, 200, 218
methicillin-resistant *Staphylococcus*
    aureus   see MRSA
metronidazole
  administration 212
  clinical indications 212
  side effects 212
  use 212
miasma theory 27
microfibre 86
microorganism
  growth cycle of 15–16
  routes of transmission 28
miliary tuberculosis 22
monobactams
  administration 202
  clinical indications 202
  use 202
Moraxella catarrhalis 208

MRSA 1, 62, 76–77, 89, 114, 163,
189–190, 200, 203, 205, 207,
209, 210, 211, 212, 215, 225
myasthenia gravis 206
mycobacteria 21–22
Mycobacterium
fortuitum 140
kansasii 22
tuberculosis 22, 31, 54
mycoplasma 207

N

National Patient Safety Agency 5, 72
necrotising fasciitis 28
needlestick injuries 29
Neisseria
gonorrhoeae 29, 35, 198
meningitidis 202
spp. 198, 208
neoarsphenamine 194
Nightingale, Florence 2, 10
norovirus 51, 52, 188
incubation and symptoms 52
prevention 52
treatment 52
Norwegian scabies 62

O

obligate
aerobes 13
anaerobes 13
occupational health 48
occupationally acquired
infection 49
Orthomyxoviridae 53
osteomyelitis 37
oxazolidinones
administration 209
clinical indications 209
use 210

P

parasites 33
Pasteurella multocida 198
pathogens
activities of 28
Patient Environment Action Team
(PEAT) 84
pelvic inflammatory disease 204
penicillin 194, 195–196
clinical indications 198
extended-spectrum 199
reaction to 199
spectrum of activity 200
spectrum of use 198
V 198
Penicillin chysogenum 195
perinatal transmission
of infection 35
personal protective equipment (PPE)
118–120
pest control 139
pharyngitis 28
Plasmodium 24
Pneumocystis jirovecii 212
poliomyelitis 49
Porphyromonas spp. 198
pre-employment health checks 48
pressure sores 36
Prevotella spp. 198
prokaryotic cells 11
prostatitis 204
Proteus spp. 139, 207
protozoa 15, 24, 33, 34
Pseudomonas 13, 202, 207
aerinosa 139
aeruginosa 21, 30, 199, 201, 202,
204, 213
spp. 21, 199
puerperal sepsis 29
pulmonary TB 189

Q

quinupristin/dalfopristin
  administration 209
  clinical indications 209
  use 209

R

reflective journal 5
Rickettsiae 207
RIDDOR 66
rifampicin
  administration 211
  clinical indications 211
  side effects 211
  use 211
root cause analysis 231

S

Salmonella 19, 51, 135
  typhi 19
Sarcoptes scabiei 61
Saving Lives tool 229
scabies 61
  incubation and symptoms 62
  preventionm 62
schistosomiasis 35
secretions 122
septicaemia 17–18
Serratia marcescens 139
sexually transmitted disease 204
sharps
  disposal 55
  injury 55
  management of 123–124
sharps/needlestick injuries 56
  post-exposure prophylaxis 57
Shigella 19
shingles
    see varicella-zoster virus
skin infections 60

smallpox 194
specimens
  management of 122
Spongiform Encephalopathy Advisory
  Committee (SEAC) 98
staff
  absence 49
  sickness 49
standard
  cleaning 82, 87
  precautions 113, 185
Staphylococcus 17–18, 194
  aureus 139, 198, 201, 203, 205, 209,
    210, 213
steam cleaning 86
sterile
  equipment 160
  service department 98, 108
sterilisation 73, 74, 105
sterilisers
  bench-top steam 105
  bowl and instrument 105
  porous-load 105
storage
  of instruments 107
strep throat 28
Streptococcus 17–18, 194, 198
  agalactiae 18
  pneumoniae 18, 201, 205, 211,
    215
  pyogenes 18, 28, 209
Streptomyces 207
  griseus 195
  roseosporus 210
  spp. 206
streptomycin 195
sulphonamide 194
surgical wound infection 36
surveillance 231
swine flu (H1N1) 53
syphilis 35

T

tetanus 21, 49
tetracyclines
administration 206
clinical indications 206
side effects 206
use 206
Tinea
corporis 23
pedis 23
tissue necrosis 21
Toxoplasma gondii 34
transmission
modes of 35
transplacental 35
transport
of instruments 107
Treponema pallidum 35, 194, 206
Trichomonas vaginalis 34
trust boards 226–227
responsibilities of 229
tuberculosis 49, 89, 189
incubation and symptoms 54
prevention 54
treatment 54
typhoid 19
Typhoid Mary 50

U

ulcers 36
ultrasonic cleaners 103
uniform 118
universal precautions 113
ureidopenicillin 199
urinary
catheters 169–176
checklist for ongoing care 175
infections 39, 204
key points to prevention 172

V

varicella–zoster virus
incubation and symptoms 61
prevention 61
treatment 61
vector-borne infection 33
ventilation 88
key points 90
systems
cleaning and maintenance of 89
viruses 15, 23

W

washer-disinfectors 103
waste
disposal of 128
segregation of 128–129
water coolers 140
best practice 143
winter vomiting disease 52

Y

yeasts 14